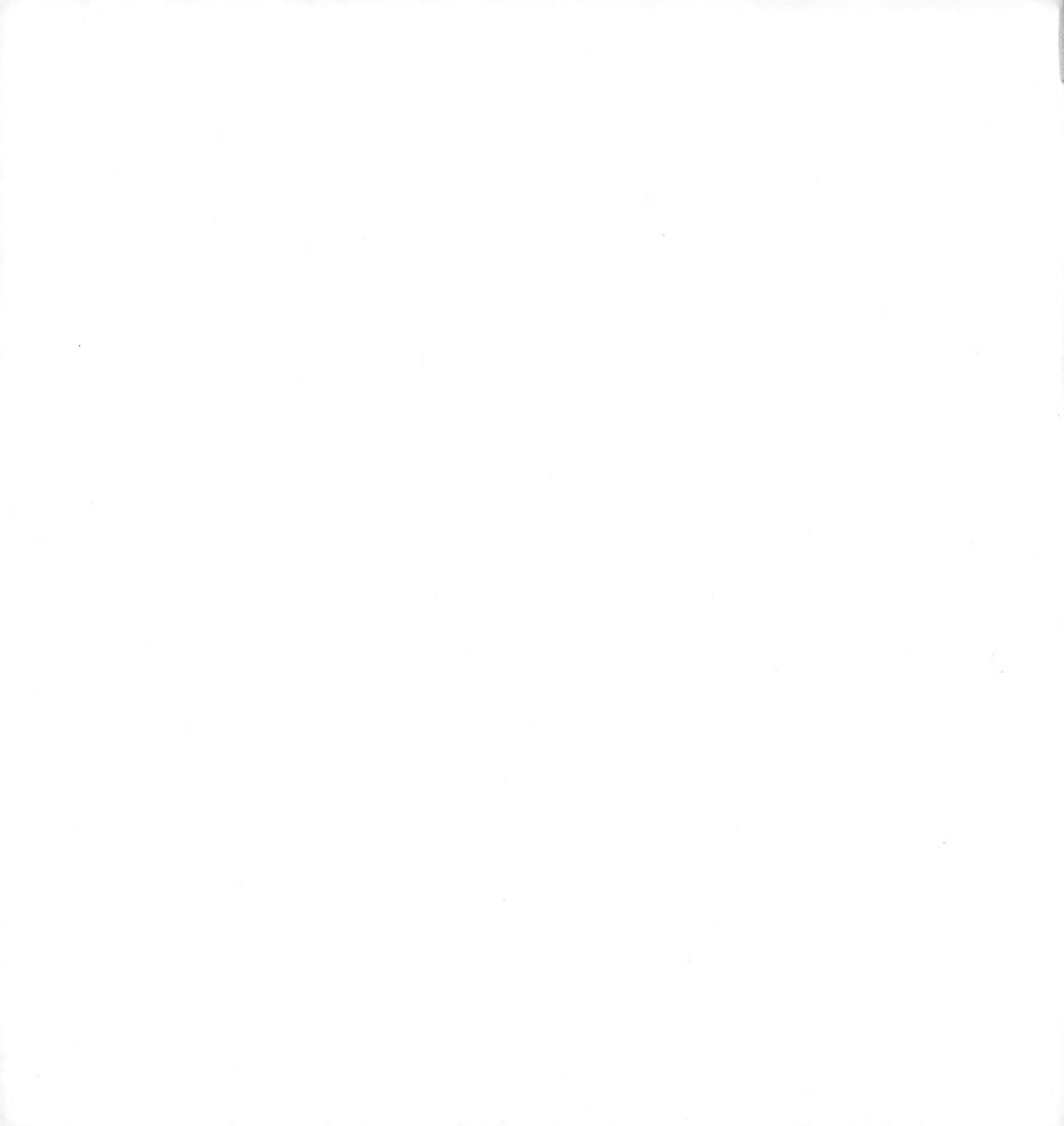

Corinna P. Kromer

A Mediterranean Infused Cookbook & Memoir

Seasonal & Allergen Free Cooking

By Corinna P. Kromer

Growing Field
Where children go to grow

"Corinna P. Kromer, A Mediterranean Infused Cookbook & Memoir"

Corinna P. Kromer, A Mediterranean Infused Cookbook & Memoir
LCCN 2020946274
ISBN: 9780985705770

Editor - Corinna Kromer
Photography by Corinna P. Kromer, Vassiliki Silira and Freepik: www.freepik.com
Cover/Page Layout by Vassiliki Silira, vassosilira@yahoo.gr

Printed in Colorado 2021

"Let food be thy medicine and medicine be thy food"

"Hippocrates"

Colorado, 2021

Corinna's cooking and her creations bring elegance to the kitchen that is centered on a Mediterranean foundation that is naturally allergen free. This cookbook provides a platform for health, based on the richness of the Mediterranean diet and shares the benefits of a seasonal approach to cooking that takes advantage of the bounty of nature. If you love Greek food and are also suffering from gluten and dairy allergies, this cookbook is filled with tasty, adaptable, everyday recipes you can make at home that are authentic and healthy. You too can explore this book today; expand your culinary repertoire and nourish a healthy state while learning from one of the best – a must have for your kitchen!

Yannis Dokos

Chef de Cuisine, Hellenic Executive Chefs Federation, Member of Euro Toque Greece

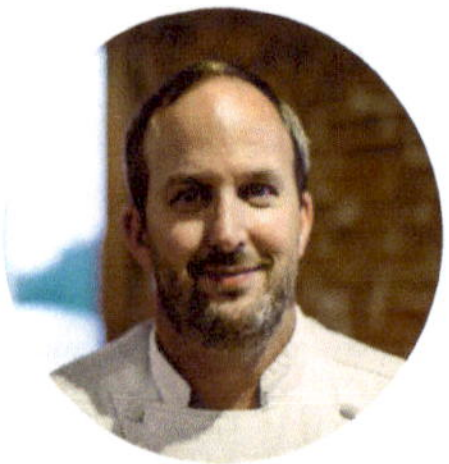

I have known the Kromer family for 12 years and was very excited to hear of Corinna's cookbook venture. Knowing the passion for food that Corinna and her husband Brian share, this book shines with delicious and health conscience dishes I've experienced from their kitchen for years. The recipes she has created in this cookbook reminds me of when we cook for the Kromers at our restaurants, good, clean flavors with seasonality in mind. Corinna's Greek heritage and family recipes provides a mindfulness as she lays out a plan for a healthy and happy life.

Jason Shaeffer

Owner/Chef, Chimney Park Restaurant & Bar, Hearth Restaurant & Pub

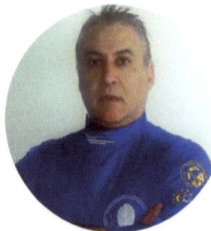

Table of Contents

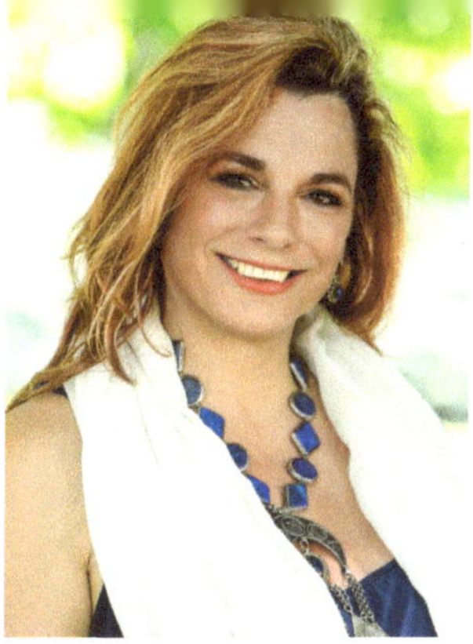

Corinna P. Kromer

Note from the Author

Welcome!

There is one question that everyone asks me when they find out about my Greek heritage, and that is "Where can I find some good authentic Greek food"? And in all the years of teaching cooking classes, sharing meals with friends and catering events, I have always been pleasantly met with the same request, "Can you make your dishes available for sale or teach us more ways of cooking Mediterranean food?" So finally, I am excited to share some wholesome and easy Mediterranean Recipes from my repertoire with you. My family and I enjoy these delicious recipes daily and hope you will as well.

There are a lot of great cooking methods and special ingredients that have been passed down to me from my Greek heritage that make these dishes delicious, full of flavor, and that are prepared with love. Most of my earlier years were spent in Greece where I grew up.

My firsthand experience of these wholesome, tasty recipes comes from spending years of watching my mom and grandma cook and from enjoying many delicious meals while spending time in the kitchen surrounded by family. Our own kids loved being in the kitchen from a very young age and enjoyed learning how to make food from simple cookies to the complicated dish of rolled grape leaves.

Growing up around the kitchen was a cherished gift for me; and my goal is that by passing those recipes down to you, along with the importance of the "cooking ritual", it will bring equal joy to your household.

Over the years I have come to learn and understand even more about nutrition and how important home cooked meals are to our health. It has also become clearer to me why the Greek way of cooking is so supportive to our health and have come to acknowledge the building blocks of a good diet. In my opinion, good diet not only promotes good health in the body, but also helps with mental health, emotional wellbeing and general wellness of our soul. Henceforth, the fresher our diet is the better we feel.

In Greece it seems everything revolves around food and company often gathers around the kitchen table. If you have ever had the good fortune to be invited over by a Greek family, you will notice that not only are they warm and hospitable, but they will always offer you a "meze" as we call them, a little edible treat, coffee, or something to drink. They will sit down with you and spend time connecting and catching up, as if you were old friends.

It is that personal connection and the feeling of having your soul nourished that I am wanting to share with you in this book; in hopes that the warmth of our culture seeps through every recipe you try.

You will notice that there are quite a few pictures in this book, some of them really old, before digital imaging, and some of Greece and of our family, not necessarily relating to a recipe. I wanted to share some of the colorful dishes and fun memories from our family and introduce you to the richness of the Greek and Medi-

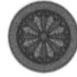

Note from the Author

terranean cuisine. You will also notice that some recipes are less involved than others. My goal was to make this a resource for all levels of culinary explorers. Some recipes will take a bit more time and are geared more towards those who like to spend extra time in the kitchen. For the most part however, I kept it fairly simple and with a Mediterranean flair.

My husband and I enjoy teaching cooking classes and sharing our knowledge of food with everyone who is willing to listen. We continuously talk about the importance of eating "clean" foods from wholesome local and organic sources and why it is important to eat with the seasons.

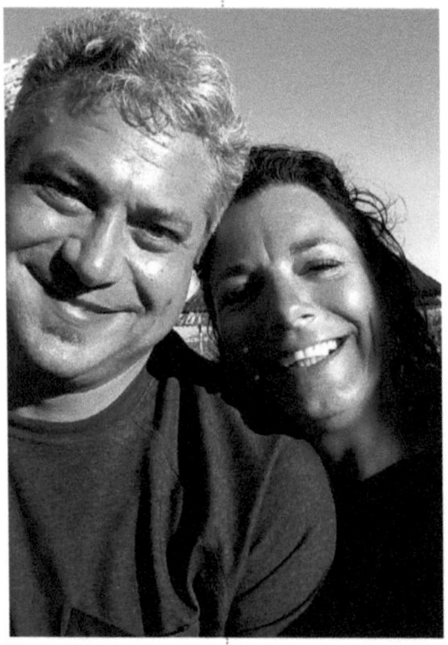

Every fruit and vegetable has a special time when it grows, ripens, and when it is harvested during the year. With the introduction of greenhouses, as well as opening the borders and shipping foods from across the world, the necessity and habit of eating with the seasons has been lost and a lot of this knowledge has disappeared.

I do believe that food provides more complete nourishment and has more life force when it is fully grown and harvested at ideal seasonal times. That is after it has absorbed enough nutrients from the earth, warmth and energy from the sun and before it finds its way to our kitchen and eventually our plates.

It is therefore important to strive and eat produce that is fresh, grown under the sun and locally available during each season, if we want to receive the optimal nourishment & vitality from our food. For that reason I have added a small note at the bottom of each recipe that denotes what season each recipe is best suited. Down the road I would like to also invest some time in writing a cookbook that is specifically dedicated to eating with the seasons.

Keep in mind, that depending where you live, your growing season for certain fruits and vegetables might be different as the climate changes from location to location. Not all veggies and fruits grow everywhere so you can make the choice of using imported foods, depending on your taste buds and preferences.

Generally speaking, you will notice that produce is more affordable when in season, as it is plentiful that time of year and might not even need to be shipped in. That is often a good indicator of what is in season or not.

Organic and home grown foods are mainly free of pesticides and chemicals. They provide our body with the

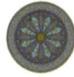

Note from the Author

delectable taste without the extra unwanted toxins that most of conventional produce is often grown and infused with. One way to get fresh organic produce is by visiting your local farmer's market, by growing your own vegetables and fruits in your garden, or even in pots inside and outside your home and garden.

The importance of mindfulness, and how our mood and emotions affect everything in our lives, including how and what we eat, is something to keep in mind as well. It is my belief that when we prepare a meal, our emotions and state of being are infused into our dishes. A recipe cooked with passion, excitement, laughter and under happy circumstances will have that special ingredient of lightheartedness infused in it and make it even more delicious!

Cooking is more than just a physical act; it is a collective body, mind and spirit experience. The ingredients and how they are grown and harvested, the recipe and its execution, eating in a peaceful and pleasant environment, and taking time to enjoy your meal, are all an important parts of how our body receives the food, accepts the nourishment and fulfills an emotional part of ourselves.

While this cookbook is just an introductory guide to Greek and Mediterranean Cooking, and some of my favorite recipes; when you pair it to the other courses, cooking events and workshops that I offer over the year, it becomes a powerful tool for growth and transformation.

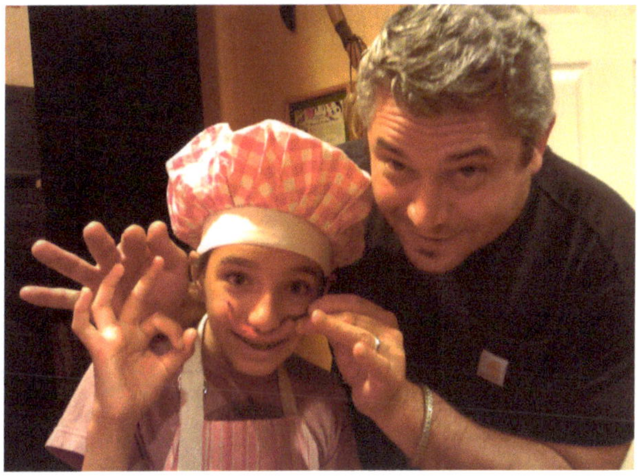

If you would like to follow events, forums and additional material available, you may join our Mediterranean Community explorations at:

www.HealthAwarenessCoach.com

YouTube videos –Corinna P. Kromer– You are invited to take a moment and visit our YouTube channel where we are slowly adding videos on mindfulness, meditation, cooking and other joyful explorations of how to live life.

When you subscribe to our channel, you will automatically get notified of all new videos as they are uploaded. Our cooking classes are slowly being added, as well.

In joyful and nourishing spirit.

Corinna P. Kromer

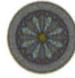

How it all began...

Gathered around the kitchen, enjoying family dinners and passing down these customs from generation to generation is a practice that is almost extinct in our time. The importance of gathering and sharing a nutritious meal is one that we have strived to keep alive in our family. As the kids reached their teen years, it became increasingly challenging to meet at the kitchen table on a regular basis. We still do share delectable meals and gatherings together however, to satisfy our craving for family time.

At the island of Crete with my Dad, my hubby, and my second Mom, after another satisfying meal

The kitchen table has seen many a conversation, has gathered family, friends, sports teams, cooking classes and even people we did not know at times... all in the name of a wholesome nutritious meal and a great time. We still spend most of our time in the kitchen, whether we are cooking, creating or sharing our latest news with family and friends.

It was not until I moved to another country in my early twenties that I began realizing how precious and rare this lifestyle is. The knowledge that has been passed down to me through life experiences is pure gold. Not only because of its nourishing values, but also because of the effect that it has in our mood and overall wellbeing. The exposure to all kinds of fruits and vegetables, seasonal growing, farm life, gathering and harvesting and spending time in the kitchen, have all been instrumental in developing my passion for good healthy food. When I was a kid, I remember being annoyed at not having tomatoes available in the winter and lettuce in the summer; but my mom would remind me that every vegetable has a season.

My passion for salads started back then, when I was disappointed that I could not have a nice, juicy tomato in the wintertime. Back then I do not remember being able to get produce from another country; so we grew and ate what was seasonally available. It took me a while to understand the importance of "eating with the seasons".

Certain vegetables thrive in the summer; others do well in the winter and the cold weather. It is the law of nature. You can bet that a tomato grown in a greenhouse in the winter time will have nowhere near the nutritious value or the taste than the one grown outside... sun kissed during the summer months. Have you ever smelled a handpicked tomato? Have you gotten a whiff of that earthy, green smell as the stem bends to separate

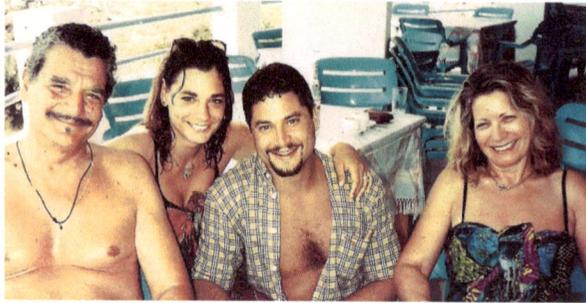

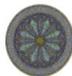

How it all began...

from its fruit and you savor the flavor of the tomato as you separate it from its vine?

You can't help but get lost in the aroma of fresh picked strawberries and other juicy, plum berries... or hear the cracking of the stem as you snap off a fresh zucchini from its plant. Your senses become alive when you pick a fruit fresh from the field or tree. Often you can experience that same fullness of that freshness in the produce available from your local farmers. My mom tends to her own organic farm and sells her produce at the local farmers market but alas she is in Greece and I am in the U.S.

I love to visit our own local farmer's markets. Thus I spend time in each farmer's stand, experiencing and smelling the freshly harvested goods before I put them in my basket and get inspired for my next meal. That is the beginning of my connection with the food, as my brain swirls with prepping and cooking ideas of how to use this "pot of gold" I just acquired. Often instead of looking for ingredients to my recipes, I let myself be guided by what is available and looks fresh at the market that day. If I see a beautiful firm eggplant, I might get inspired to make a juicy "Imam Bayildi", a Mediterranean vegetarian dish with onions, bell peppers and tomatoes that is so good it melts in your mouth!

Unfortunately, in today's world, where boxed and frozen foods and canned fruits and vegetables abound, the knowledge for pure, natural food and how to prepare it

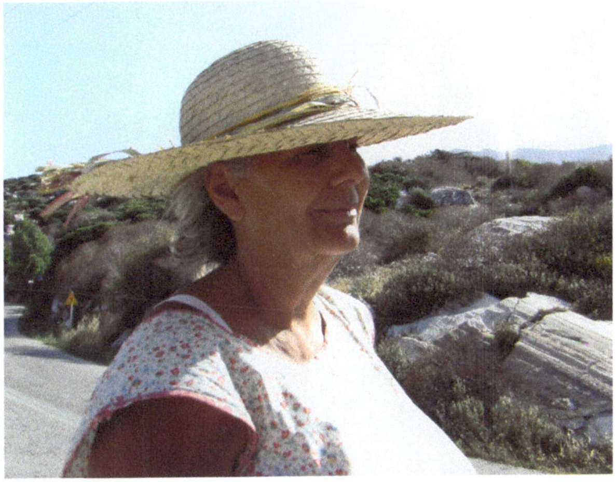

My beautiful & creative Momma

is becoming more and more scarce. It is also for this reason that I decided to compile a few of my favorite recipes in this book. I would like to thank my many friends who have constantly been nudging me to share some of my favorite flavors and "how to" instructions with them. I am grateful for their queries and support as this has been a task to undertake, but well worth it.

Some of these recipes are old Greek and Mediterranean classics that have been passed down generations. Others are recipes I have been inspired with over the years that my family enjoys. If you would like to follow the seasons and try out some simple recipes from scratch, not only healthy but also delicious, I invite you to explore this book

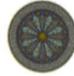

How it all began...

With my second dad

from cover to cover and have fun with it. There is no right or wrong way of using it. Just go where you are called and you are sure to fall on a tasty gem.

This book has been divided into several sections of foods and every recipe is listed under that. You will notice that at the end of each recipe, there is a note about what season this recipe is best enjoyed. That is because you are more likely to be able to find those ingredients fresh at that time of year, and get the best nutrition and taste out of it.

Each recipe is also marked for certain allergies and diet preferences, and they are marked as gluten free/vegetarian/dairy free. Our family has had its own challenges over the years with allergens, and I have learned to adapt just about any recipe to suit our complicated needs. Currently, we are avoiding gluten, dairy and soy products and after much practice, about 90% of our recipes follow that directive.

These symbols on the top left & right of each recipe will guide you to those:

Vegetarian: V   Gluten Free: GF

Dairy Free: DF

My husband, my children and I, travel to Greece each year to visit our family and friends, immerse ourselves in the culture and enjoy delectable local foods. I hope through this book you too can travel to Greece with us, enjoy the local tastes and get a sense of the rich and nutritious Greek and Mediterranean cuisine.

Thank you for the opportunity to share my culture and experiences with you. May your taste buds awaken and your senses be tantalized!

Στην υγειά σας! - To your health!

Corinna P. Kromer

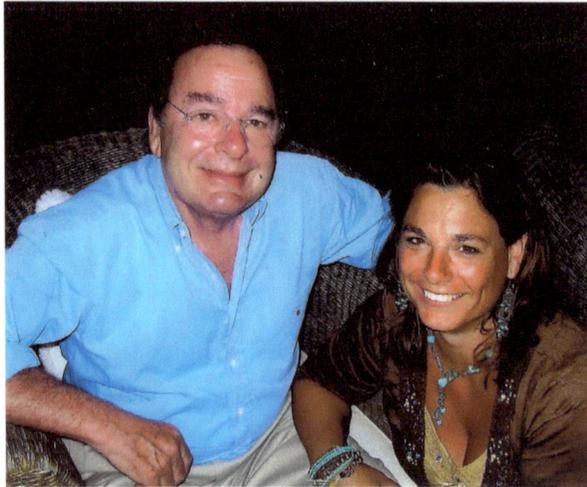

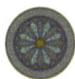

A platform of Health

In this section I will cover some essential ingredients and staples in the Greek and Mediterranean Cuisine with a little bit of background information to get a feeling of how we use them. Some other unique foods that Greece is known for are honey, salt of the sea, wild and healing herbs, select fruit and of course, many of it's cheeses.

Cheese: White and yellow cheeses are commonly available in Greece. One of the most well-known is Feta cheese, and I am sure you have probably heard of it. Originally made from sheep's milk, it is a brined cured white cheese that is known around the world for its particular taste.

A Greek "village" salad, called Horiatiki in Greek, is not complete without a big slab of feta cheese, sprinkled olive oil and oregano on top. A very unique taste, it will vary substantially in taste from north to south and east to west.

This cheese is so popular that other countries have tried to imitate its taste and warm up to its palate. In the United States it is usually made with cow's milk, and alas, it does not at all taste the same or have the same texture. So if you are looking for the original experience, make sure the feta you buy is made from sheep or goat milk or a mixture thereof. There are also other unique yellow cheeses that one might compare to Italian varieties such as Kefalotyri, Graviera and Kasseri. Kefalotiri is a hard, aged cheese similar to Parmesan or Romano cheese and is used for grating over pasta or in Saganaki, which is

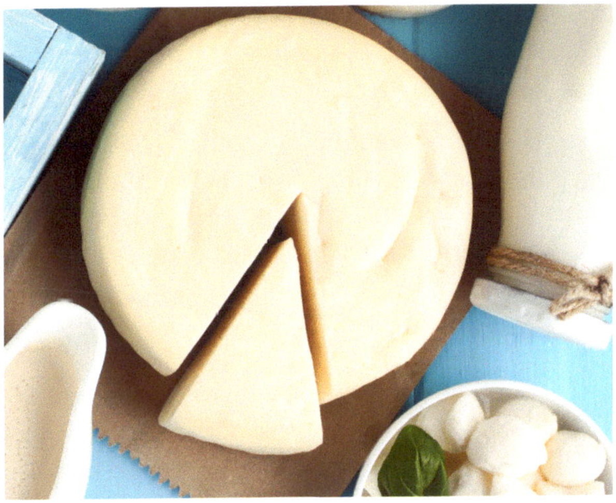

fried cheese. The salty, piquant taste of kefalotiri comes from aging; which must be for at least 3 months to be considered a true kefalotiri cheese.

Graviera cheese is one of the most popular cheeses in Greece. It's a hard cheese with a light yellow color, and it has a slightly sweet and nutty taste. Its salt content cannot be greater than 2 percent. Kasseri cheese is a Greek sheep's milk cheese with a rubbery texture and a sharp, salty flavor. Kasseri is a good melting cheese. This cheese is also well known as the cheese used in the Greek dish called Saganaki. There are also other popular cheeses such as Mizithra, similar in taste to Ricotta cheese, Ladotyri, which is made from ewe's milk and has a strong taste and is very tasty in salads. Also, there

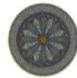

A platform of Health

is Manouri cheese which is a soft, creamy cheese from Macedonia, with a subtle taste and often used in dessert and pie recipes.

Each one has its unique bouquet and pairs well with several Greek and Mediterranean dishes. While some cheeses are complete without brine or salt preparation, others need to be immersed in the brine and aged allowing for a unique and more flavorful experience.

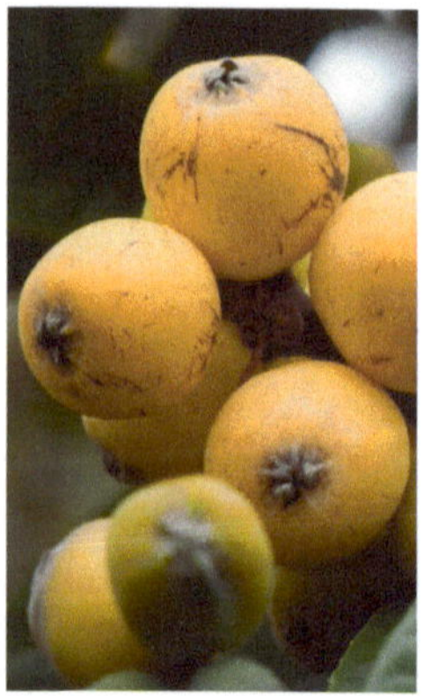

Fruit trees and groves are spread out and in abundance. Some of the juiciest peaches you will ever have the pleasure of tasting are grown in Greece. You will also find grapes, oranges, mandarins, apricots, figs, loquat and many more. Kiwi groves – a later addition to our climate - are found in areas of the country as well. Sweet bananas, also grow mostly in the southern islands where it is a dryer and warmer climate. Tasting a fruit that is in season is like an explosion of heaven in your mouth. Strawberries, mulberries and boysenberries are abundant as well and can be found out in the wild or in local neighborhoods.

Fish and Seafood: Since Greece is surrounded by water, cod, sole, red mullet, mackerel, tuna and other less common fish are a big part of the diet. Octopus, squid, and shellfish are also popular, and play a large part in the Greek cuisine. As you can imagine seafood is high in iodine, an important element for our health; which is probably one of the reasons why the Mediterranean diet is so healthy for body and mind.

Iodine is required for healthy thyroid function, the regulation of metabolism, cell reproduction and absorption of oxygen, and also helps keep our nerve function at its optimum level. In the United States it is estimated that most of the population is Iodine deficient, causing thyroid issues, weight fluctuations and problems with many of our glands. Regularly adding seafood to your diet can help bring more balance to your system.

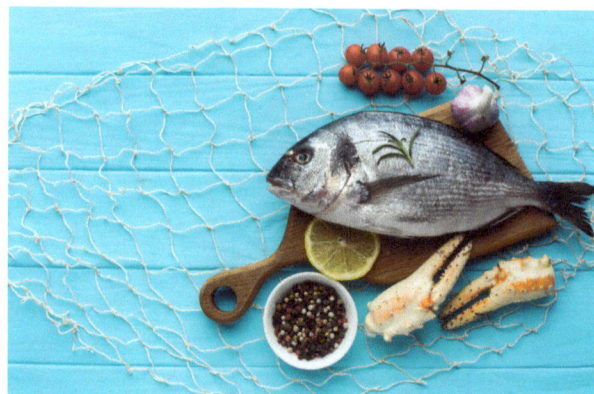

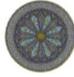

A platform of Health

Fish is often flavored with bay leaves, rosemary and thyme and is served with a dressing of fresh olive oil and lemon juice.

Herbs abound in the hills and mountains of Greece wherever you look. In my walks around nature, I easily spot wild thyme, wild sage, mountain tea, oregano, helicrysum and St. John's Wort.

Capers grow wild on my mother's farm and my father's island home. Oregano, laurel leaves, helicrysum, dill, fennel, mint, marjoram, rosemary, saffron, and many other gifts from nature can be found or grown to be used in cooking and for remedies. Besides using herbs and plants for cooking, I really enjoy having a variety of herbs in our garden. From those, I make my own potions and lotions, from beauty and hygiene products, to natural remedies.

Every year when I travel back home to Greece, I hike up the mountains and on islands and gather fresh local herbs that I then dry and use in the kitchen for cooking and for DIY recipes.

Often, I will make burning incense sticks from wild sage gathered from the hills of Paros, a Greek island of the Cyclades. When I burn the sage it smells heavenly. Everybody loves its slow burning, pungent and cleansing attributes. Herbs are sustainably harvested taking care not to stress the plant or its future propagation qualities.

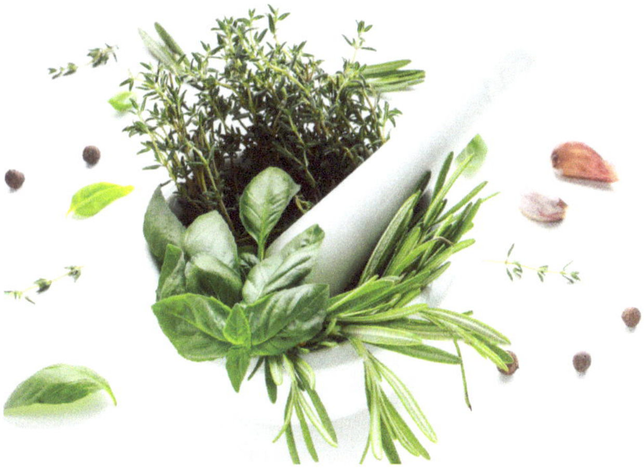

Naturally, each herb needs to be picked at its prime time and season for the fullest flavor experience.

Climate changes often affect the end product, as different geographic locations in Greece are humid or dry, warmer or cooler, mountainous or by the ocean front. The same herb can taste very different depending where and when it was harvested. No matter where they are picked, their taste and aroma is a welcome addition to our daily dishes.

Honey abounds in Greece and again, you have a different taste depending where it is harvested. Some bees will feast in orange groves, others on flowering thyme bushes and sometimes they enjoy lavender and wildflowers.

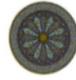

A platform of Health

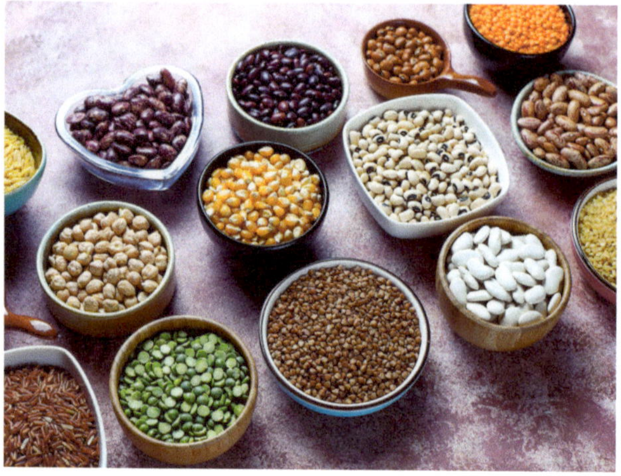

Most honey is deep in flavor and thick in viscosity. Honey has been adored since the ancient times and has been known as the food of the "Gods". It is a daily staple in our kitchen, and I use it in cooking, baking, tea making and home remedies.

A spoonful of raw honey will cure your sore throat and make you feel better. If you have allergies, consuming raw local honey can help build your immune system, relieve inflammation and help you get relief from environmental sensitivities. It is a subtle and healthy sweetener for drinks, baked goods and sauces.

Legumes: Legumes are a great addition to any cooking, not only for their abundant nutrients, but also for the delectable taste. It is always best to use dry beans instead of canned, but that is your preference. If you are using dry legumes in your recipes, such as chickpeas, kidney beans or black eyed peas, make sure to soak the beans overnight to make them more easily digestible.

Lentils do not need to be soaked ahead of time but do need to be rinsed as dirt and little pebbles can be present in the mix. Pour out two cups of your preferred legume (usually a recipe's worth) in a large bowl, cover with enough water and then let them soak for at least 8 hours.

Take into account that as they absorb the water, they take up more space, so make sure your bowl is large enough.

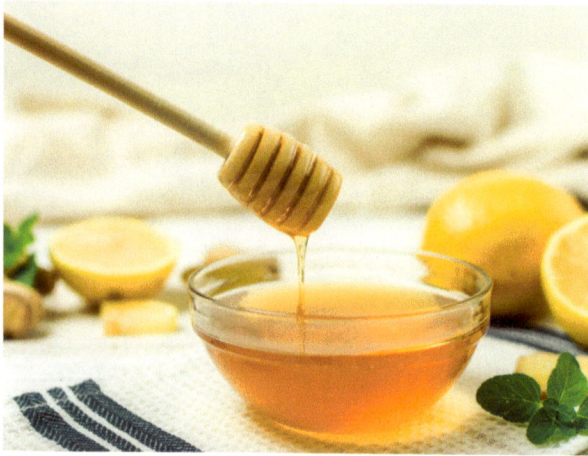

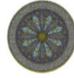

A platform of Health

Check on them half way, as sometimes they might need extra water added. Some people like to use the liquid in which they are soaked to cook the legumes, and others prefer to use clean water or broth. Some of the nutrients will remain in the water when you soak them, but for people who have a more sensitive digestion system, it is usually better to discard the soaked water. Most legumes need a long time to cook, at least an hour but if you do not mind using a pressure cooker, it can cut your cooking time substantially.

Nuts: In general, the harvesting of nuts happens in the autumn/winter season. However, nuts such as almonds, walnuts, filberts and cashews can be stored for a long time and be used throughout the year for different recipes.

Chestnuts are an exception, as they need to be cooked when fresh. – Either roasted or pressured cooked, they do not tend to keep for long periods of time. However, they can be found in the market processed, either canned or boiled.

Almonds, walnuts, and chestnut trees grew in our yard when I was growing up. I remember sitting on the ground with my best friend for hours cracking and eating the pine nuts that fell on the ground from the pine trees. Nowadays, you can purchase chestnuts raw, dry, boiled or roasted, processed in foil bags or even cans.

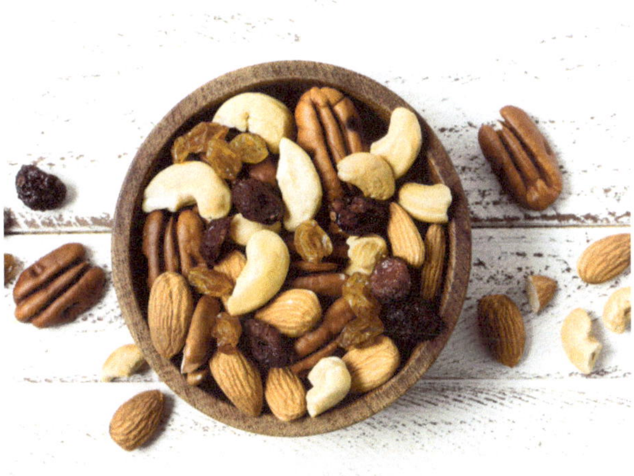

The taste, as with everything else is not the same as when they are fresh. Many nuts such as the chestnuts, are only available seasonally during the winter months. To keep nuts fresh, make sure to store them in airtight containers or freeze them.

We love to eat nuts raw with some cheese and/or honey, sprinkle them in our salads and even add some to our yoghurt with a bit of honey on top. Beneficial oils such as omega 3, 6, 9, unsaturated fats, fiber, vitamin E and the amount of protein in nuts make them a healthy and quick snack. Research suggests that eating nuts may lower your bad cholesterol and triglyceride levels, improve the health of the lining of your arteries, lower levels of inflammation linked to heart disease, and re-

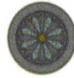

A platform of Health

duce the risk of developing blood clots. As a result of adding healthy nuts to your diet, I have read that this can improve your heart health and lower your risk of heart disease, as well.

Olive oil: When we think of Greece and Mediterranean Cuisine we think of Olive oil. Olive oil is the cornerstone of the Mediterranean diet, perhaps the healthiest in the world. Studies have shown that olive oil lowers "bad" cholesterol and cuts your risk of heart disease, stroke, and cancer of the breast, prostate, and colon. It eases joint pain without side effects. Authentic, high-quality olive oil is an antioxidant rich superfood that lowers inflammation, is cardio- protective, and improves gut health.

Olive oil is delicious, has zero carbs and makes recipes more flavorful. As one of the healthiest fats, it keeps us full and satisfied long after meals. It keeps snacking to a minimum because of that. Indeed, this is one of the most wholesome ingredients used in this culture, and an essential ingredient in most recipes. Nowadays, I tend to add a bit of coconut oil, ghee and fresh butter to my repertoire, but the original flavors and health benefits are derived from the usage of pure, cold pressed olive oil.

If you have visited Greece, you will have noticed the abundance of olive groves available throughout the land. To this day, there are still some olive trees that date back more than a thousand years and that boast a trunk several feet wide. These trees have been part of the Greek land from as far back as 3,000 B.C. Olive oil trade was common between Egypt and Asia Minor even back then.

Olive trees have always been considered a blessing in this part of the world and the stories that surround it date back to mythical times. According to legend the olive tree, considered to be the most useful offering to mankind, was given to the humans as a gift by goddess Athena. In ancient times olive wreaths were used to crown the winners of the Olympic Games and amphorae filled with olive oil were given as a prize to game winners. Olive oil was rubbed all over the body in ancient days

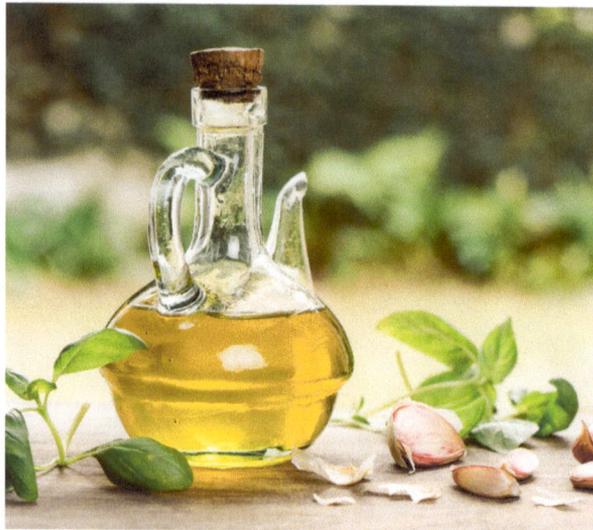

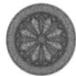

A platform of Health

as it was believed to be rejuvenating for the skin and expressed good health and vitality.

An olive tree wreath was also hung on a door to announce the birth of a child. To this day olive oil is still widely used in cooking, baking, making breads and sauces. It is also used to make soaps and other natural hygiene and self-care products. A spoonful of olive oil is still often consumed first thing in the morning as a preventative measure, and it is believed that it is essential to the proper inner workings of the body.

Olives are another staple in the Greek and Mediterranean cuisine, often eaten as a snack or as an accompaniment in salads and spreads. Greece produces an abundance of different types of olives. Probably the most well-known are Kalamata olives and Throumbi olives; a wrinkled variety that comes from the island of Thassos, but there are many more. Greek olives are generally very strong in flavor and have a deep pungent taste to them. Most olives need to be fermented and processed before consumption; as they are typically very bitter when fresh. Salt, vinegar & herbs and sometimes olive oil itself is used to age the fruit.

Often you will find them for sale in barrels and large containers where you can buy them in bulk and by weight.

When choosing an olive, the fruit should be firm and balanced in taste where you can taste the olive over the brine.

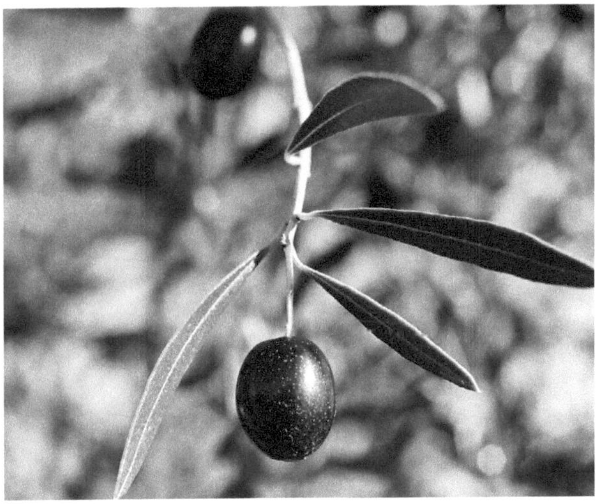

Traditionally, most types of olives are harvested in the late fall, when the fruit is ripe and full of its juice. Some olives will be put into brine for several months and become a delicious treat and some will be used to press and produce the precious olive oil. During the months of October, November and maybe even December the hustle and bustle is prevalent as villagers rush to their fields to collect the fruit. Even those who live in the city will take some time off to go harvest their beautiful crops. My mother, has several olive groves, and typically heads out around late October to go north and check the abundance that is awaiting collection. Many fields are still harvested by hand.

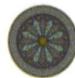

A platform of Health

Huge tarps and nets are laid down under and around the trees to contain the olives as they are knocked down with long sticks, taking care to not bruise the fruit. There is nothing like the taste of the homemade olive oil. Each year I bring back some olive oil from home, to dress a salad and gently cook a meal in.

There are three varieties of olive oil: extra virgin, virgin and pure. The less the oleic acid present in the final product the better the flavor.

The best olive oil is extracted when the olives go through a cold press process (no heat is used to extract the liquid). The highest quality oil then comes from the first cold press of a healthy crop of olives.

Pure olive oil is the lowest grade made of the second and third pressings of the olive, and where pits, skins and the pulp of the remainder from the first and second press are used. Pure oil may be often mixed with virgin oil to give it the flavor that has been lost through the process.

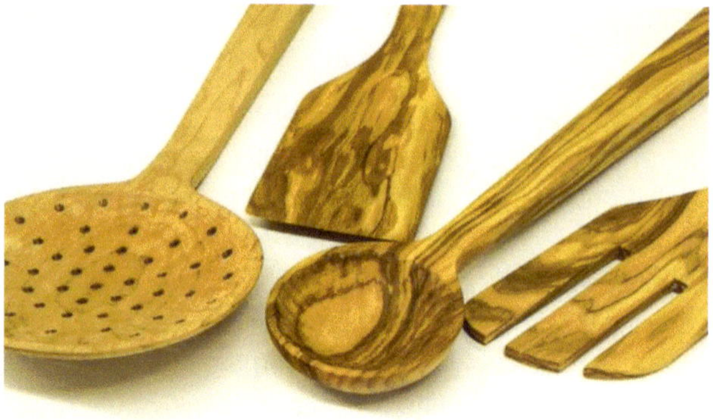

When buying olive oil, I always look for a rich, dark olive green color, a delicious full smell and I take note of the viscosity of the product by feeling it between my fingers. I don't like my olive oil to be too runny; instead a nice thicker, fuller weight is preferable. Olive oil should be stored in a dark, dry place. Usually a glass or metal container is best to prevent aging and oxidation.

Olive wood creations: When a tree is uprooted by a storm or just no longer lives, its wood will have many uses. Often in the Greek markets you will see kitchen utensils made out of the sturdy wood that comes from olive trees. Bowls, cutting boards, decorative items and even sometimes older furniture can be found that are made of good quality olive wood.

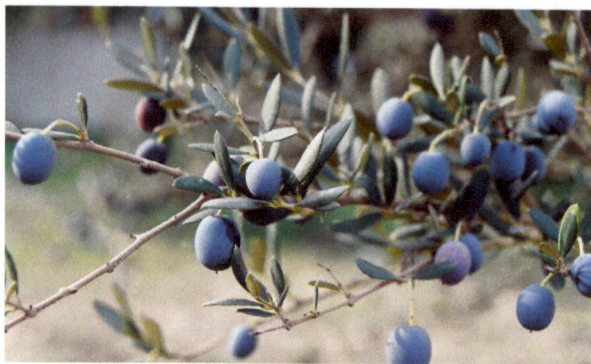

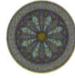

A platform of Health

Sea salt is harvested in many areas in Greece and is generally very salty tasting (unlike some Tibetan sea salt varieties) and is full of minerals and nutrients such as Iodine. You can often find it raw and unfiltered in its crystal or flake form. It is delicious for cooking and also for curing meats and storing foods.

Sea salt comes in different coarseness, depending on what you need to use it for. Coarse salt can be used while cooking a meal, while finer salt is usually reserved for use at the dinner table and topping salads and appetizers. Different qualities and flavors of salt can be used to accentuate your own palate.

The items below are some of the main staples that I keep in my kitchen on a regular basis and are mentioned in this cookbook frequently. Many of the Greek recipes are elaborate and will call for a few of these ingredients, but I did try to keep this cookbook fairly simple. If you enjoy this type of cooking, you should consider keeping those on hand. The list is alphabetically and not in order of importance in the Mediterranean cuisine.

Mediterranean & Favorite Staples	
Bacon Fat	Lemons
Bay leaves	Lentils
Butter, Yellow or plant based	Mayonnaise, plant based
Bread	Kalamata Olives
Bread Crumbs, regular or GF	Olives
Chickpeas, dry	Olive Oil
Eggplant	Onions, yellow & red
Eggs	Organic Vegetable Shortening
Feta Cheese	Pepper, cracked
Flour, regular or GF	Pine nuts
Freshly cut veggies (carrots, cucumbers, celery, jicama, lettuce)	Salt, raw from ocean
Garlic	Vinegar, red wine
Herbs, Basil, Marjoram, Oregano, Rosemary, Thyme	Vinegar, Apple cider
Honey	Yoghurt, Greek - strained

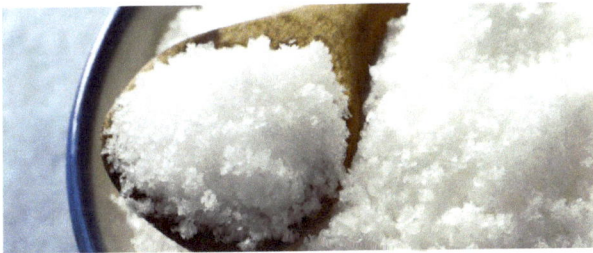

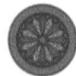

Additional Info - Substitutions

Baking: Unless otherwise stated, all of my baked recipes are prepared in a **convection oven and at high altitude.** If using a conventional bake oven setting, times might slightly increase as convection ovens are normally more time efficient. You can search online for conversion times and schedules. Baking in high altitude tends to add cooking time to a recipe, so if you are at sea level cooking times might be slightly less (about 10-15 minutes depending on the recipe).

Butter/Dairy Free options (DF): If you prefer to avoid dairy, you may substitute organic vegetable shortening, usually with a ratio of 1:1. Nowadays, there are a number of vegetable spreads available that are dairy free and soy free. Olive oil, however, is a great and healthy substitute in many recipes. It is my experience that complicated, non-dairy alternatives sometimes have additives which are not healthy for your body, and I prefer using simple fresh solutions, such as coconut oil, olive oil or even nut oils.

Gluten Free (GF): If a recipe calls for wheat flour or thickener, I have discovered that gluten free flour (usually a mixture of rice, quinoa, potato/tapioca starch) substitutes well on a 1:2 ratio. Due to the lack of gluten, you will need more GF flour to mix for the same recipe. As far as making roux or thickener, that will depend on how thick you like your sauces, but in general, I have found it to be a 1:3 ratio. There are a few gluten free baking mixes out in the market that are very palatable and work well in most recipes. However, I urge you to check the ingredients, as most premade gluten free flour mixtures have added ingredients such as sugar, molasses, inulin, salt, etc. I prefer the ones that are simple mixtures of flour for my cooking, but that is up to you. If you are handy and like to mix your own flour for a gluten free experience, you will need a heavy base such as quinoa, mixed in with either brown or white rice flour and a starch; either potato, amaranth, or tapioca works well to make it more fluffy and light and easily digestible.

The lack of a starch can make a recipe very dense and hard to eat. If you like to experiment in the kitchen, you can play around with different flour mixtures to find your favorite flour taste and weight. One gluten free combination that I have used often is 2 cups of quinoa flour, mixed with ½ cup of potato starch and ½ cup of arrowroot starch.

Milk/Dairy Free (DF): In any recipe that calls for milk/cream ingredients, I have often substituted either almond or coconut milk. One of my favorite substitutes is organic coconut cream, which lends a full and smooth taste to most recipes requiring a touch of dairy. Canned coconut milk in general gives a much richer and wholesome taste, and the coconut taste is not too strong. If you need to keep dairy out of your diet, feel free to switch those out while still keeping the integrity of the recipe.

Many of the almond milk options in the market also have a lot of sugar in them, as well as flavoring. While those might be an easy alternative for coffee or tea, I have found a couple of very simple products in the market

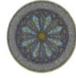

Additional Info - Substitutions

that only contain a few ingredients and no sugar for my baking and cooking needs. Always beware of alternative sources of milk that are full of additives such as sugar and other added ingredients which are not necessary.

It is a matter of taste though, so I invite you to try out several options and find the one you like best.

Pressure cooker: If you have a busy schedule and time is an issue, in preparing fresh meals for you and your family, a pressure cooker can save you a lot of time. While I am not aware of any negative aspects of cooking your foods this way, it is possible that one may lose some nutrients when subjecting the food to this type of cooking. Legumes however, such as dry chickpeas, beans and soy can often take more than 90 minutes to fully cook, but the time can be reduced to a few minutes by using a pressure cooker.

For someone with a busy schedule that still wants to cook wholesome meals, that makes a big difference. Adding a teaspoon of oil in your pressure cooker will help in reducing frothing as the food cooks and to avoid clogging your pressure topper. It might be helpful to remove the froth first as you begin to boil the legumes and then seal the pressure cooker to continue the cooking.

One of my family's favorite dishes is chicken soup. It takes just 15 minutes to pressure cook the whole chicken, and not only is it delicious for a cold winter night, but it also happens to be beneficial for our immune system. So if you feel the sniffles coming on it is one of the best remedies. Just make sure to use a whole (organic) chicken, bones and all. You might find that a pressure cooker will become your best friend for some of your more involved dishes.

Sugar: Whenever you see reference to sugar I refer to **organic raw sugar.** You may also substitute with coconut sugar or white cane sugar according to your preference. I have found that many of our domestic sources for beet sugar are not to my liking and standards, as they contain a lot of toxins. I prefer to use more wholesome options. Often you can substitute honey or even maple syrup in your recipes.

Abbreviations

lbs. *pounds*

tsp. *teaspoon*

tbsp. *tablespoon*

V *Denotes Vegetarian Recipe*

GF *Denotes Gluten Free Recipe*

DF *Denotes Dairy Free Recipe*

Ω *Wherever applicable, I have added the Greek name of the dish for your perusal and fun. It is in blue at the top of each recipe.*

Recipes

I

Wholesome Great Starters

BREAKFAST

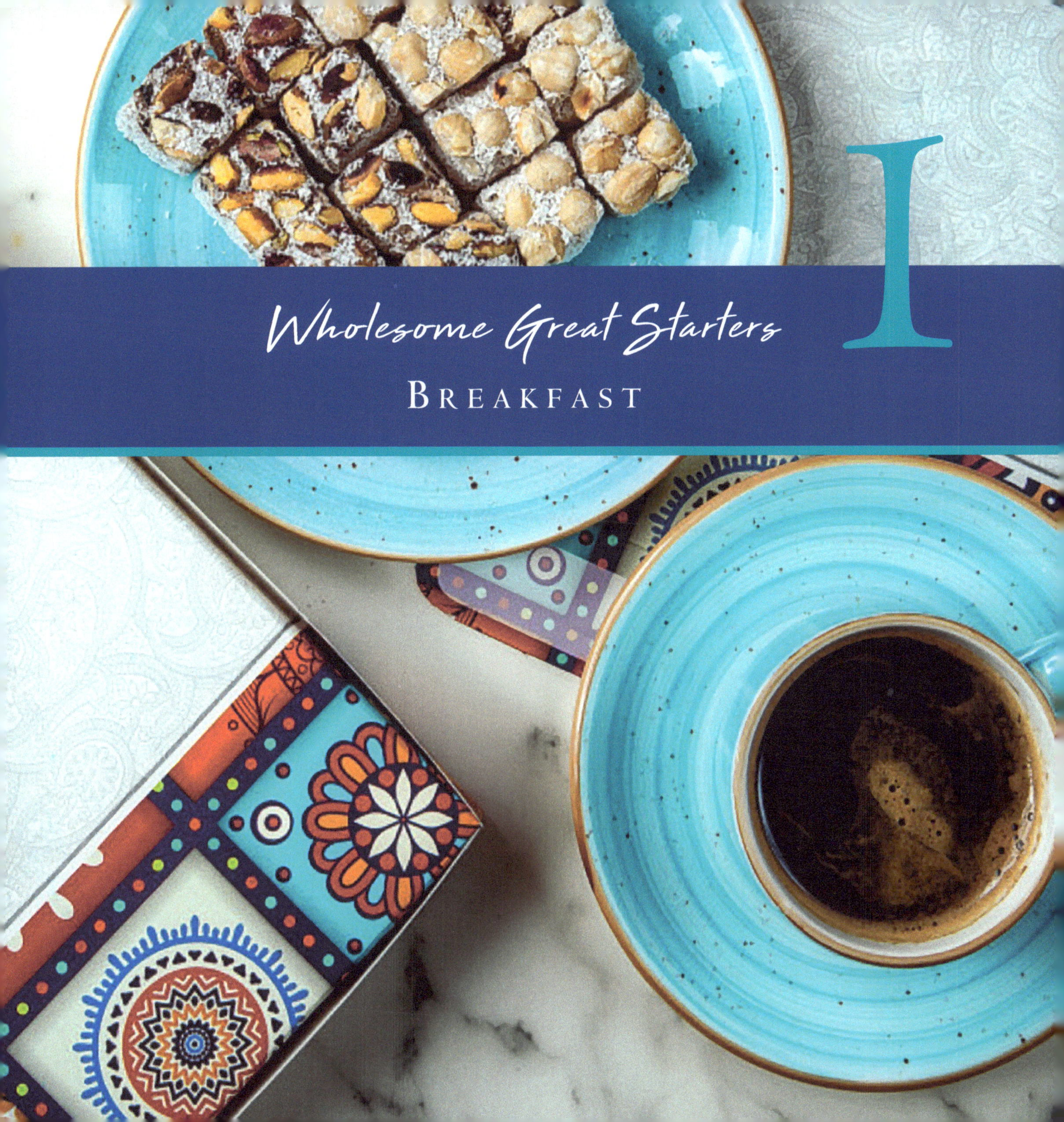

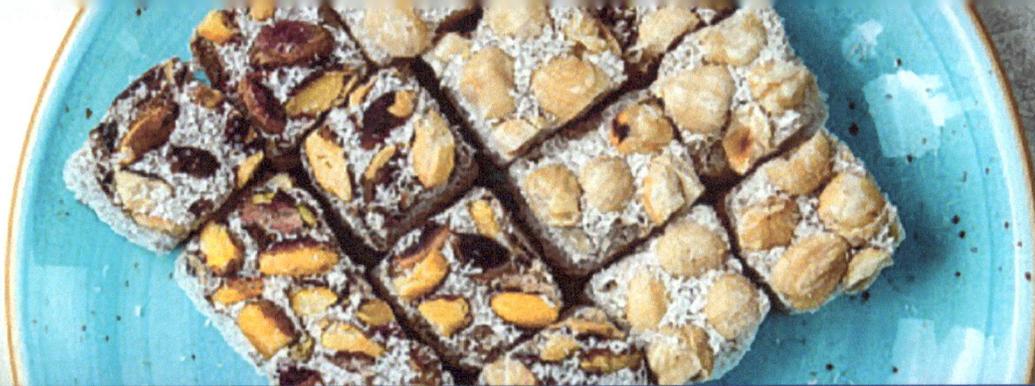

DF GF V

Wholesome Great Starters - Breakfast

Apple Chicken Sausage Frittata

This is a super easy and fast cooking morning recipe. Apple chicken sausages are one of our favorites, and I thought I would add it into a frittata and see what it tastes like.

It turns out it is delicious, and has become one of our new favorites! I like to use sources of sausages that are all natural, without artificial ingredients or use of antibiotics.

This recipe can be perfect year round but the tomatoes will be tastier during the summer months.

- 2 tbsp. olive oil
- 1 package of pre-cooked apple chicken sausages, sliced in rounds
- 4 green onions, sliced
- 10 fresh eggs
- 8 cherry tomatoes, halved
- 1 cup shredded yellow cheese of your preference
  - Avoid Salt as the sausages are salty enough
  - Pepper to your tasting
  - Parsley sprigs for garnish if you like

Preheat oven to 375° F.

Place olive oil and sliced sausages in a heated iron skillet (that can go in the oven). Gently sauté the sausages until they start browning and then add the green onions for about a minute.

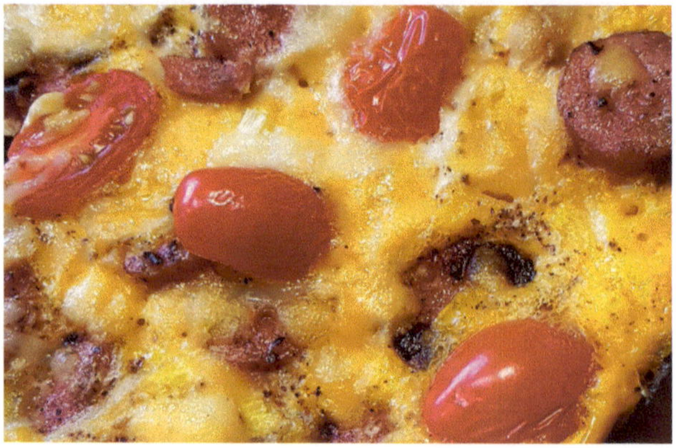

Crack eggs into a bowl – although I do not like to mix my eggs as in an omelet, I always crack the eggs in another container, one by one to make sure they are fresh.

Add eggs into the pan with the sausages and gently swirl them around with a spatula, breaking the yolks but not mixing them too much. When the eggs begin to whiten on the bottom and are half cooked, sprinkle the cherry tomatoes on top. Add the shredded cheese and pop the pan into the oven for about 8 minutes.

Keep checking the oven and when the eggs are cooked and the cheese melted, remove the pan from the oven and let it rest on the stove for a couple of minutes.

Serve warm like a pizza slice and enjoy the aroma of a fresh frittata.

Serves 4-6 people *(All Seasons)*

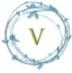

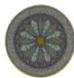

GF DF

Bacon Onion Quiche

One morning I woke up with a craving for quiche. Anyone who follows a gluten free diet knows how disappointing it is to be at a restaurant where they serve a delicious quiche and not be able to try it. So I came up with my own recipe below. Since I am temporarily (I hope) dairy free as well this tasty recipe is made with coconut crème.

You will notice that this recipe calls for bacon fat. This is a staple in our kitchen and I use it for many things that may call for butter or oil. Just drain the fat from when you cook bacon and save it in the freezer.

For the crust

- 2 cups organic blanched almond flour
- ½ cup bacon fat
- 1 tsp. sea salt
- ½ cup chopped yellow onion
- ½ cup dairy free shredded cheese (Reserve another ½ cup for the top crust)

Filling

- 8 eggs, whipped together
- ½ cup coconut crème
- ½ cup chopped yellow onion
- ¼ cup finely chopped chives
- ½ cup dairy free cheese shreds (or regular shredded cheese)
  - Salt + pepper to taste

Preheat oven to 400° F. In a medium bowl mix together almond flour, sea salt, onions and bacon fat and blend well until mixture is somewhat pasty but still crumbly. Layer out the pastry in a round pie baking dish and push around with your fingers until the crust evenly covers the bottom of the dish and 2/3 up its side.

It is ok if it is a bit uneven, as long as most of it is spread out. Bake the pie for 8 minutes and take out to cool.

Meanwhile mix together the eggs until well blended, add salt, coconut crème, onion, chives and cheese and blend well. Add pepper if desired. When crust has cooled down, add filling to the pan and put back in the oven under the same temperature for 15 minutes. Check quiche and if browning too fast on top, bring down temperature to 350° F for another 20 minutes. Check doneness by inserting a fork in the middle of the pie. If it comes out clean, your pie is ready. Sprinkle extra cheese over crust and give it another 5 minutes in the oven. Remove from oven and let rest 10 minutes before serving. Enjoy!

Serves 8 people *(All Seasons)*

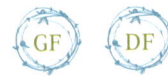

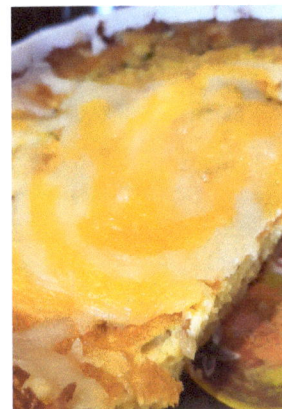

GF

Corinna's Breakfast Bowl

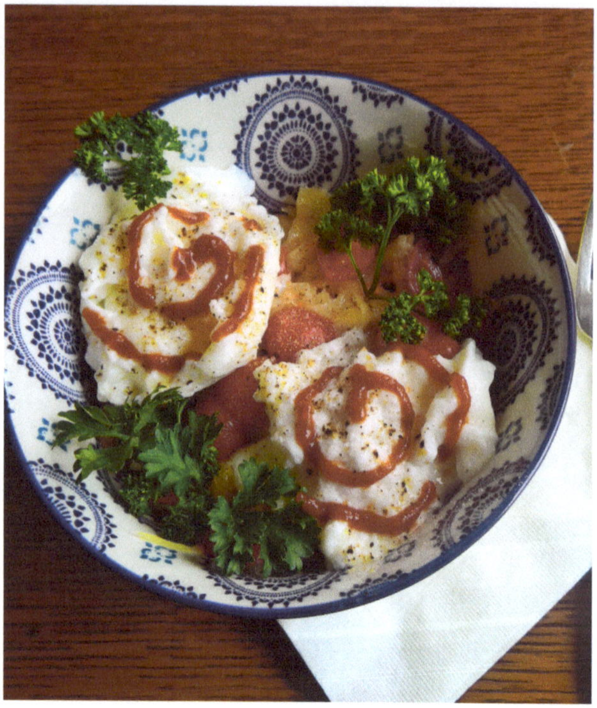

This was a creation that came about one morning as I was thinking of what to do for breakfast, and saw the left over baked potatoes from the previous night's dinner. Left over tater tots are another good base that has worked really well with this dish.

Perfect year round.

3 large baked potatoes, cubed

5 slices of ham, shredded or cut up in small pieces

1 cup shredded Jarlsberg cheese

2 cups cherry tomatoes, halved

8 poached eggs

4 finely sliced green onions for garnish

2 tbsp. hot sauce to drizzle on top

- Salt + Pepper to your tasting
- Parsley sprigs for garnish

Preheat oven to 300° F.

In a large ramekin, layer about 1 cup of baked potato cubes on the bottom, then top with shredded ham, Jarlsberg cheese and cherry tomatoes and put in oven to bring to warm temperature.

Meanwhile poach 8 eggs to medium, where the yolk is still runny in the middle and lay on top of cherry tomatoes in the warmed up bowl. Top with green onions, salt, pepper and sprinkle with hot sauce to your liking (or omit altogether). Add parsley sprigs and serve.

Serves 4 people *(All seasons)*

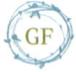

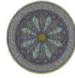

Millet & Stewed Apples

This warm and gooey breakfast helps activate the digestion process in the morning and prepare the body for the rest of the day. Perfect during fall.

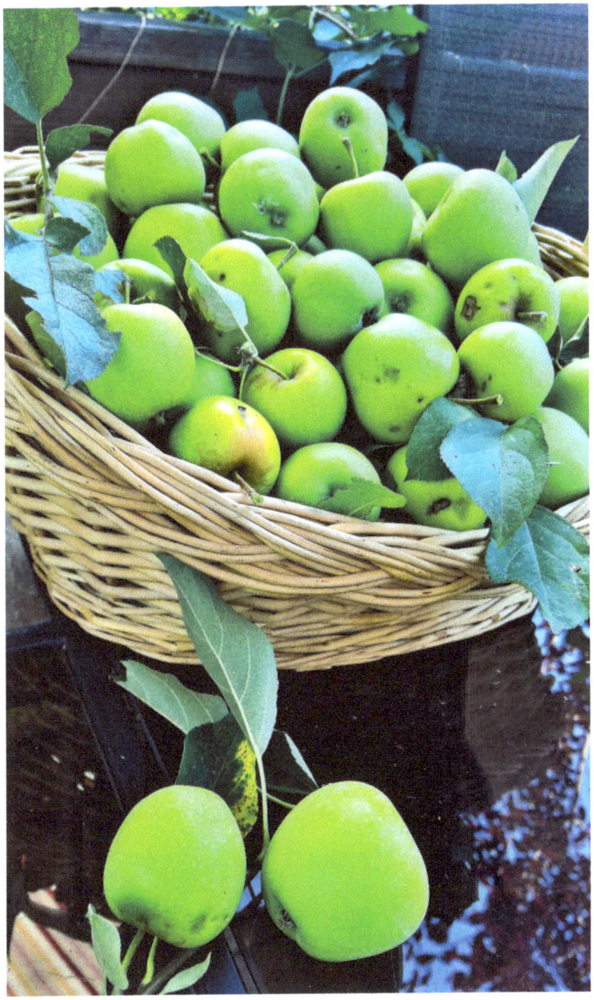

For stewed apples

1 whole fresh, red sweet apple, cored and peeled

5 whole cloves

¼ cup of filtered water

For millet

3/4 cup whole milk

2 tbsps. millet (flakes)

1 tsp. lemon juice

Dice apple into small pieces, add cloves and water and simmer in a small pot until apples are soft, about 5 minutes.

Remove cloves and discard, then remove apples from pot and cool slightly. Meanwhile add milk in pot and bring to a boil. Slowly add millet and simmer for about twenty minutes. Add apples into millet and mix. Remove to a small bowl and cool slightly before enjoying.

Serves 1 person *(Autumn, Winter)*

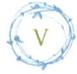

DF GF V

Wholesome Great Starters - Breakfast

Popovers with Egg & Cheese – Gluten Free

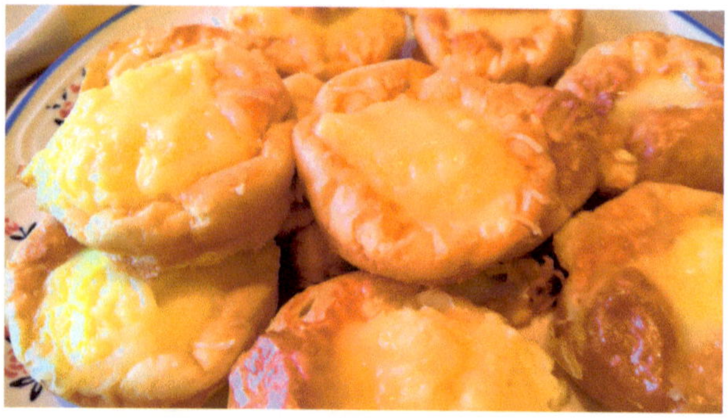

This recipe was inspired by a local bakery that makes delicious mini breakfast quiches that smell and taste heavenly. Their recipe does have wheat flour however, and it is unfortunatelly not available in a gluten free version.

So messing around in the kitchen, I came up with a gluten free version that tastes similar, and soon became a favorite in our house. Still wholesome. Still delicious. And so filling!

Gluten Free Pop Overs

- 4 large organic eggs
- 3 tbsps. melted butter
- 1 ¼ cup lukewarm milk
- 1 cup multipurpose gluten free flour
- ¼ tsp. xanthan gum
- ½ tsp. salt

Egg Filling

- 4 organic eggs
- 1 tbsp. half & half
- 1 tbsp. heavy cream (or milk if not available)
- ¼ cup shredded Swiss cheese
- 1 tbsp. shredded Parmesan cheese
- ½ cup chopped up ham or bacon crumbles (optional)
- ¼ tsp. salt (omit if using bacon)
  - Black pepper to taste (optional)
  - ¼ cup shredded Swiss cheese to sprinkle on top when cooked

Preheat oven to 400° F and grease a 12 cup muffin pan with oil or butter.

For the popovers: whisk together the eggs, melted butter, and warm milk in a large bowl. In a separate bowl, whisk the flour with the xanthan gum and salt, then gradually sift and whisk into the liquid ingredients until you have a smooth batter. Pour the liquid batter into the greased muffin pan, filing each about 2/3 full. Bake at 400° F for 18 minutes.

Fort the egg mixture: Meanwhile mix 4 eggs, half & half, heavy cream/milk and shredded cheeses (add ham or bacon if using) until well blended. Take a medium pan,

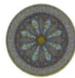

Popovers with Egg & Cheese – Gluten Free

lightly oil it and warm up to medium on the stove (just for 15 seconds or so). Then add egg mixture and barely cook while folding eggs with spatula, making sure it is still mostly liquid. Once the mixture is half solid, half runny, they are ready to be added to the half cooked pop overs. Set pan aside and off the fire.

Pull muffin pan out of the oven after 18 minutes of baking and get ready to add egg mixture. With a small silicone spatula, gently make a whole in the middle of the popovers (they will be hollow in the middle) and pour in about 1 tbsp. of the egg mixture from the pan. Once you have filled all popovers, put pan back in the oven and cook for another 8-10 minutes, until they are golden brown and egg mixture is fully cooked.

If you run out of egg mixture before you fill all the popovers, it is ok. They are just as delicious plain. But in general the above amount should be enough for all 12 popovers.

Remove from the oven and let stand about five minutes so they can firm up. Sprinkle with some extra shredded cheese if you'd like and then gently remove from pan by twirling the silicone spatula around each one and lifting. Serve on a platter. Delicious while they are still warm and gooey.

**These popovers can be frozen for about three months if you have extras. They are just as delicious when you warm them back up in the oven.*

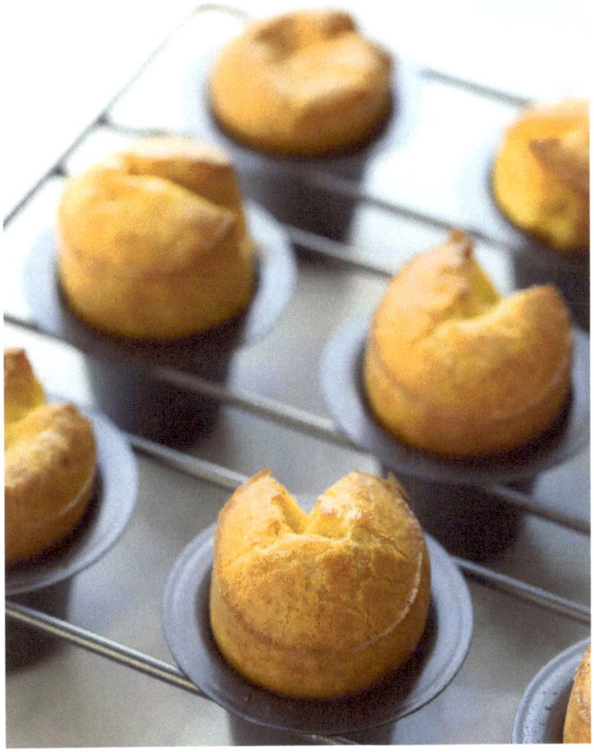

***I have had great success making these dairy free as well. I used vegetable shortening, almond milk, and dairy free cheese instead and they were delicious.*

Serves 6 people ***(All Seasons)***

- For a vegetarian version omit the ham/bacon.

Scrambled Eggs & Bacon

Eggs are considered by many to be the perfect food providing important protein and nutrients. Likewise, fat is essential to our metabolism when consumed in moderation. This is a classic continental breakfast, usually enjoyed over the weekend. The difference here, is in the way I like to cook the eggs.

My preference is to crack the eggs directly in the pan and use a soft spatula to move them around in a medium hot temperature and barely mix the white with the yellow. Feel free to add any veggies to the mix such as green onions, spinach, kale and toss with your eggs or on the side. Softer leafy veggies will cook fast and blend in easy.

For thicker veggies such as bell peppers, leeks, onions, either chop up fine to cook evenly or pre-cook by sauteeing first in the pan and then adding the eggs. Perfect for any time of the year. Hens usually slow down with their production of eggs during the colder months, so you might have a shorter supply. Did you know that a fresh egg yolk has a beautiful deep orange color?

Bread

1 slice of gluten free multigrain bread (optional)

Bacon

2 slices of natural, uncured, pork or Canadian bacon

Eggs

2-3 farm fresh eggs

1 tsp. of fresh yellow butter or olive oil

- Salt + Pepper to taste

Cook your bacon first, as it takes quite a bit longer to prepare. Either slow sizzle in a pan on the stovetop or convection bake in the oven on 300° F on a dripping pan to drain the fat.

When bacon is almost done, start on your eggs. On high heat, melt butter in pan, crack eggs directly into the pan and use a soft spatula to gently stir the eggs. Gently break the egg yolks but do not mix entirely with the white part of the egg.

Meanwhile, toast your bread to your desired crispness. Continue gently mixing & turning eggs until thoroughly cooked but not dry.

Serve bacon on bread slice and scrambled eggs on top. Add veggies on the side if desired.

**Use vegetable shortening instead for a dairy free recipe.*

Serves 1 person ***(All Seasons)***

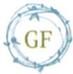

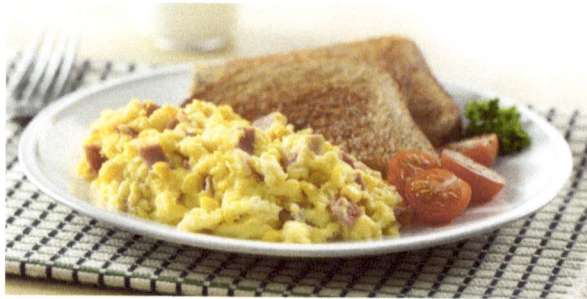

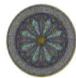

GF V

(Greek) Yoghurt with honey & walnuts Breakfast Bowl

Γιαούρτι με μέλι

Want something fast and simple but very nutritious and good for you? A quick and effortless breakfast that satisfies your palate and your tummy. My preference is yoghurt that is thick and heavy. In Greece we call "bag yoghurt" because we place it in cheese cloth and let it hang and drain for a day, allowing the mixture to become really thick.

Look for the words "Greek strained yoghurt" if you want to achieve a similar experience for this recipe. Yoghurt is a great source of protein and mixed with nuts or fruit it is a good start to your day. It is also a wonderful source of good bacteria and helps keep the probiotic population in your gut strong and healthy.

Try to use local raw honey if possible, as it is helpful with allergies and supports your immune system.

Perfect year round.

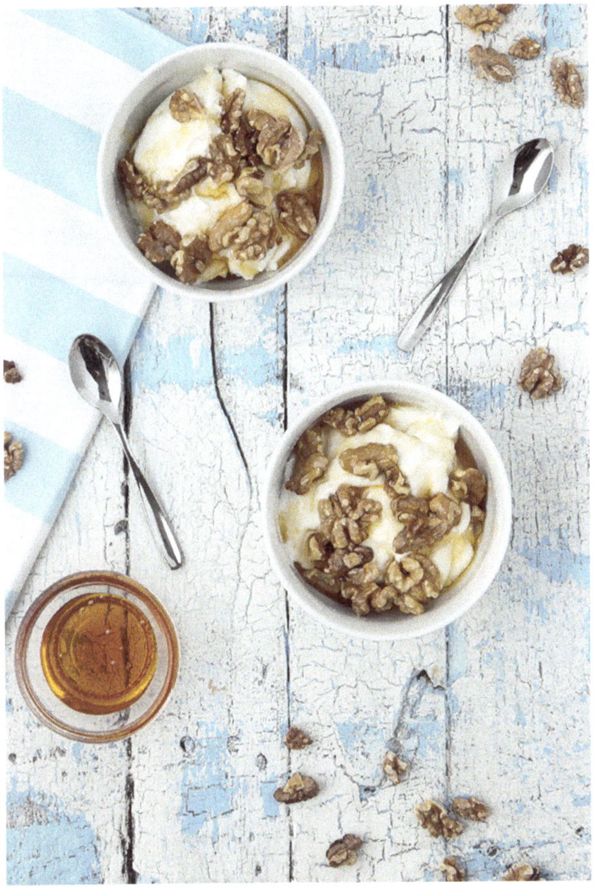

¾ cup yoghurt

2 tbsp. raw honey

¼ cup organic walnuts

Pour yoghurt in a bowl, top with honey and nuts and enjoy.

Serves 1 person *(All Seasons)*

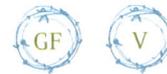

Scrumptious Squash & Onion Quiche

Unlike most quiches, this is an easy and relatively fast recipe that will tantalize your tastebuds. A special treat if you follow a gluten free or vegan diet. In autumn, squash and zucchini are abundant and sometimes continue into the winter season depending on your climate.

This is usually the time when I come up with new recipes to take advantage of the abundance of squash. And if you are not too fond of these veggies, this is a good blend that is not too powerful on the palate. Try it for yourself.

Quiche crust (bottom)

- 1 ¼ cups organic blanched almond flour
- ¼ cup organic all vegetable shortening
- ½ tsp. sea salt
- 1 large egg, beaten
- 1 tsp. minced shallot (optional)

Filling

- 1 medium zucchini, thinly sliced
- 1 medium yellow squash, thinly sliced
- 1 medium onion, thinly sliced
- 6 eggs, beaten
- ⅓ cup organic vegie broth
- ½ cup sharp cheddar cheese, shredded
- ½ cup Parmigiana Romano cheese, shredded
  - Salt to taste but optional since the parmesan is salty itself

Preheat oven to 350° F.

For the crust I like to combine all ingredients in a bowl and use my hand or a crust blender to mix all ingredients well. Or, you can put the almond flour and salt in a food processor and pulse until well blended.

Then add egg and shortening and pulse again and finally throw in the shallots, if using. Mix ingredients well until dough starts to come together and forms a ball. Then

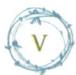

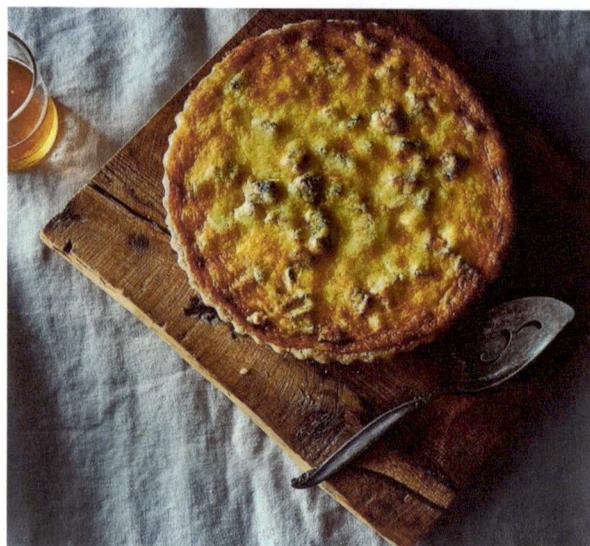

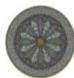

Scrumptious Squash & Onion Quiche

press dough evenly into the bottom of a 9" glass Pyrex or spring form pan with a removable bottom.

Make sure to come up the sides all the way to the rim and cover the pan evenly. Bake the crust for about 8 – 10 minutes until it turns golden and then remove from oven and let cool completely before filling.

Raise oven temperature to 425° F.

For the filling: if you happen to have a vegetable spiral slicer you may use that to thinly slice the squash and onion. Otherwise just slice each vegetable (zucchini, squash & onion) very thin and add to a large bowl. Beat together six eggs and add to the bowl. Add 1/3 cup vegie broth.

Mix the shredded cheeses together and take ½ cup of the blended cheese and add to the bowl. Blend ingredients together making sure all vegies are well coated with the liquid and slowly pour into your prepped crust. Top with remaining cheese, put in the oven and convection bake for about 35 minutes. Quiche should not have any liquid in the middle when it is done. Take out and let stand about five minutes. Cut and serve.

**Dairy Free version: even with this recipe that requires quite a bit of cheese I have made a delicious quiche with dairy free grated cheese alternatives. There is a plethora of vegan cheeses available nowadays and you can choose from cheddar to parmesan and more.*

Serves 8 people *(All Seasons)*

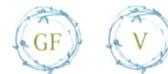

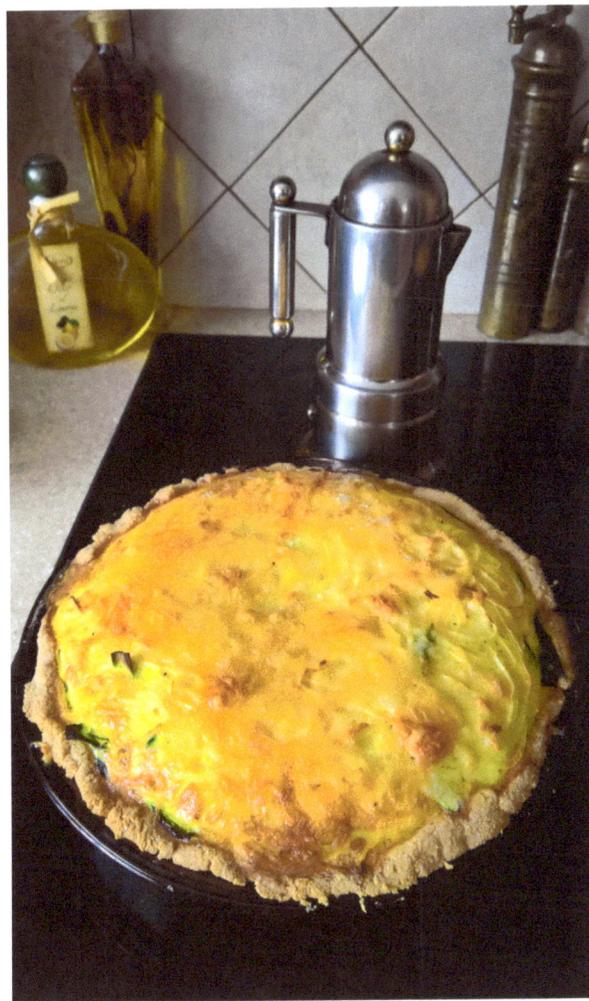

2

Great Beginnings

Appetizers & Such - Mezes (snacks)

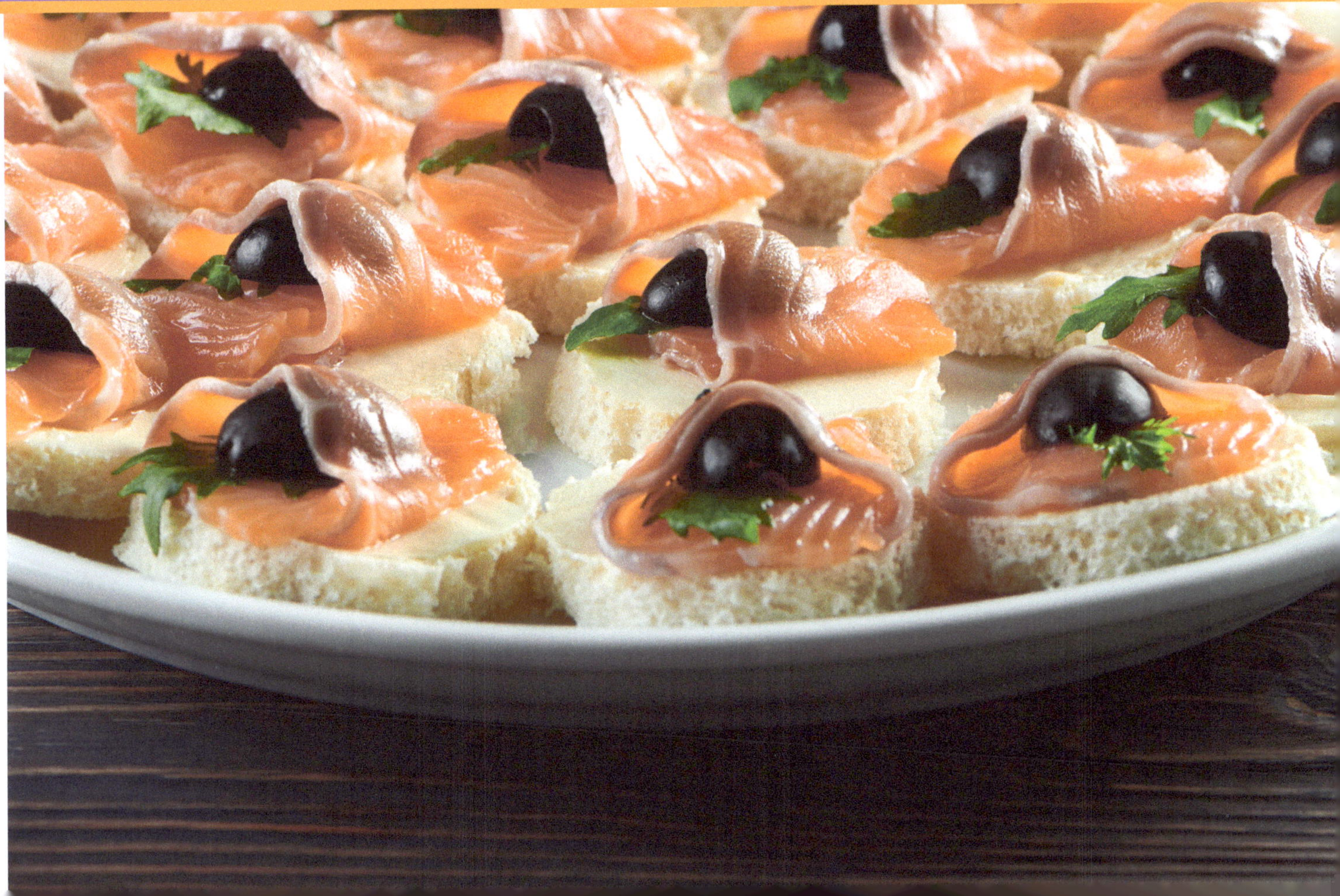

Great Beginnings - Appetizers - Mezes - Snacks

YOU ARE WELCOME!

It is a Greek custom to always serve a little something to guests that show up often times unannounced. Part of

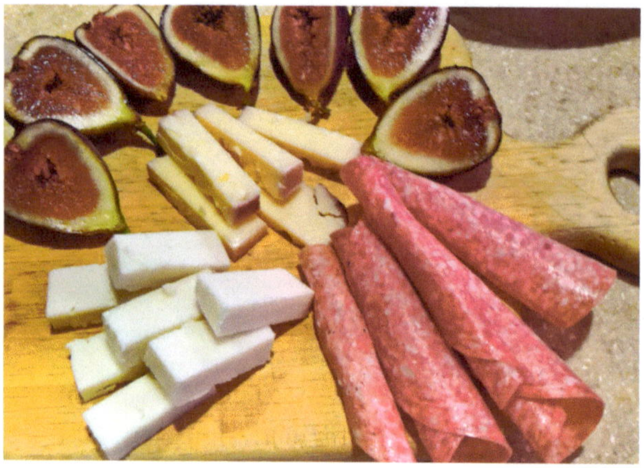

the blessing of having been brought up in Greece, was that family and friends often showed up at our house to say hello, catch up and spend some time together. Even nowadays, in our home in the U.S., friends will show up at our doorstep just for a few minutes to visit, or sometimes for a long visit. As a "good" host, we offer our guests tasty treats such as freshly baked "kouloura-kia" (cookies), some Greek coffee, Greek olives, mouth sized bites of feta cheese, some fresh bread, homemade sweets, fresh figs and other seasonal fruit and home-made delights.

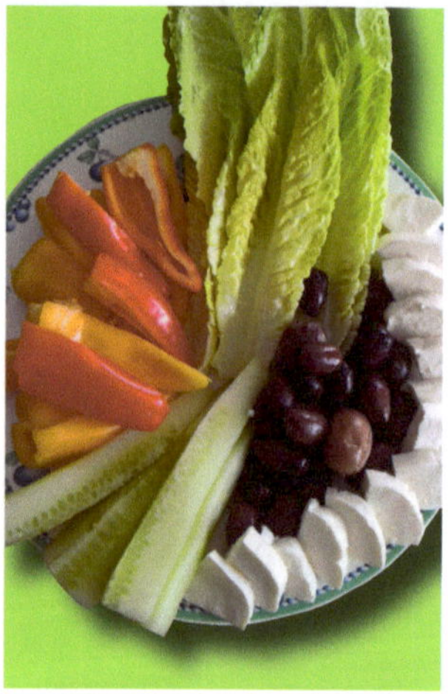

Times have changed a bit since I was growing up, but you still see the occasional grandmother sitting by the front porch in Greece, out in the sunshine, cleaning fruit, preparing beans, and spending time to create delicacies from the sea-sonal harvest. I will often find my mom sitting out on the porch cleaning beans, lentils and what-ever the harvest of the day might be. There was always something sweet or home made to share with guests in our home and to this day we carry on the same tradition at our house and always offer something deli-cious to our visitors.

If you do not have something ready, it doesn't take great effort to prepare something quick, depending on the sta-ples you like to keep around in the kitchen. For us, some of those staples include: Feta cheese and other yellow cheeses, hard salamis and charcuteries, olives, fresh bread or pitta, fresh fruit and cut up vegetables, such as carrots, celery, bell peppers or tomatoes sprinkled with a bit of olive oil and oregano. It is easy to get a quick medley together to offer with some fresh brewed coffee or tea.

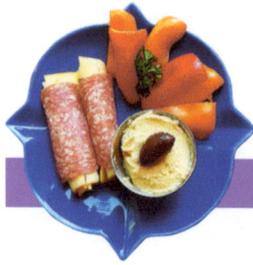

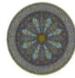

DF GF V

Crunchy Kale Chips - Collective Inspiration

This recipe came about while experimenting with different ways to cook kale while making it palatable for our young kids. I tried different spices, and dressed it in different ways and this is one of the most popular versions in our kitchen. Kids came from across the neighborhood to have kale chips when they smelled it cooking.

- 2-4 bunches of kale (Russian or Lacinato kale will do)
- 4 cloves of garlic – minced
- 2 tbsp. olive oil
- 1 tbsp. coconut aminos (optional)
  - Salt, pepper to taste
  - Other optional preferred seasonings can be ginger, garlic salt, season salt, kelp or lemon.

Soak and wash kale leaves thoroughly and tear into big rough pieces, separating from the stem, in a large salad bowl. Kale will shrink considerably when baked so use at least 2 bunches.

Toss and dress with olive oil, garlic, salt and pepper or other spices to your liking and blend well. One of my favorites is kelp or Dulce for seasoning. The saltiness of the seaweed gives it a unique taste and is full of iodine and sea nutrients.

Lay kale onto a large baking pan in a thin layer and bake at 350° F for about 30 minutes or until crisp. Check oven after first 10 minutes and turn kale over with tongues; then turn every 5/10 minutes until desired crispness is reached. Kale will turn dark green/brown but taste will be wholesome and crunchy.

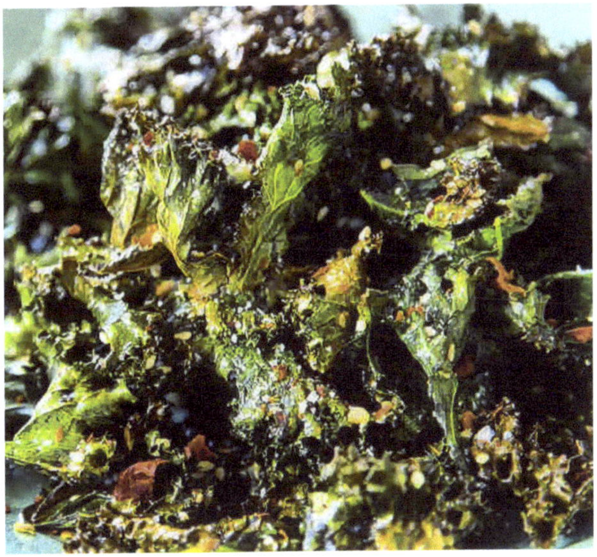

Serve into a deep bowl and enjoy as a side dish.

Serves 6 people *(All Seasons)*

Pair with: Serve as a snack or finger food, or serve with grilled salmon & roasted potatoes. Crumble the leftover small pieces of kale chips at the bottom of the pan and use as a highly nutritious spice on salads or meat/chicken/fish dishes.

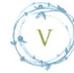

DF GF V

Great Beginnings - Appetizers - Mezes - Snacks

(Mediterranean) Hummus with paprika

This hummus recipe is one of my favorites, as it is not only tasty but also the perfect consistency. While hummus is not widely found in Greece, we do have some other dipping pastes that we make with chickpeas and beans that are also delicious. Hummus is more of a Middle-Eastern treat and is a staple in our diet, as it can be eaten in many different ways.

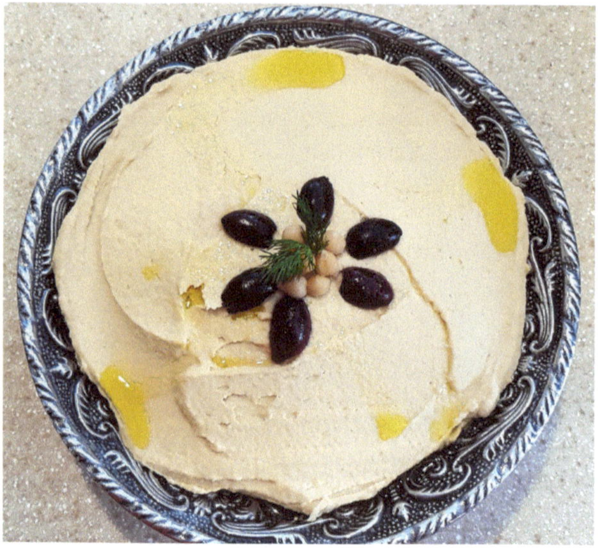

- 2 cups of dry chickpeas, soaked for 8 hours or more.
  (or two 14 oz. cans of chickpea beans)
- 1 cup of chickpea juice or water – or more according to your preferred consistency
- 2 tbsp. Tahini (sesame paste)
- 3 fresh cloves of garlic
- 2 large fresh lemons, squeezed
- 1 tsp. dry paprika
- ½ tsp. salt

For Garnish

- 1 tbsp. olive oil
  Dash of paprika
- 1 sprig of parsley
- 1 Kalamata olive, pitted

If you are comfortable using a pressure cooker, cook the soaked chickpeas until they are soft. (Your pressure cooker should come with a cooking time guide to use in each recipe). In our altitude in Colorado, I pressure cook them for 18 minutes in enough water to cover the chickpeas. Adding a tablespoon of olive oil in your pressure cooker before you seal it will help keep the frothing down and not block your valve.

Otherwise, add raw chickpeas to a large pot, cover with enough water and one tablespoon of olive oil to top the chickpeas and cook for about an hour until chickpeas are soft. If the chickpeas begin frothing, use a slotted spoon to remove the froth from the top as they continue to cook.

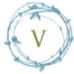

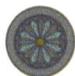

(Mediterranean) Hummus with paprika

Using a food processor, add chickpeas, the cup of chickpea broth or water, garlic, lemon juice, salt and paprika and blend until paste is smooth. I often roast red peppers and stock them in a jar in the fridge and then use them in recipes such as these. If you like roasted red peppers, the taste is richer when you use the actual peppers instead of the dry powdered spice of paprika. You can add salt and lemon to achieve your preferred taste. You might need to add more liquid to the food processor if the mix becomes too thick. You want the hummus thick enough to pick up with a carrot stick. Unless you are using it as a salad dressing, in which case you might want to make it a bit more liquid.

When the paste is smooth and your preferred consistency, serve in a bowl, drizzle olive oil and paprika powder on top and garnish with parsley and olive.

Hummus can be served as an appetizer or a side dish. You can cut up fresh veggies such as carrots, celery, peppers, or jicama and dip them into the paste. You can use it as a dip for pitta chips. You can put a dollop on your salad or even use it as dressing when made more liquid. It can be served on the side of meat dishes such as keftedakia, kebabs, lamb or fish skewers. It is really pretty diverse. Use your creativity and let your taste buds guide you.

Serves 6 people ***(All Seasons)***

Pair with: Serve as a wholesome appetizer, a side for meats, or salad dressing.

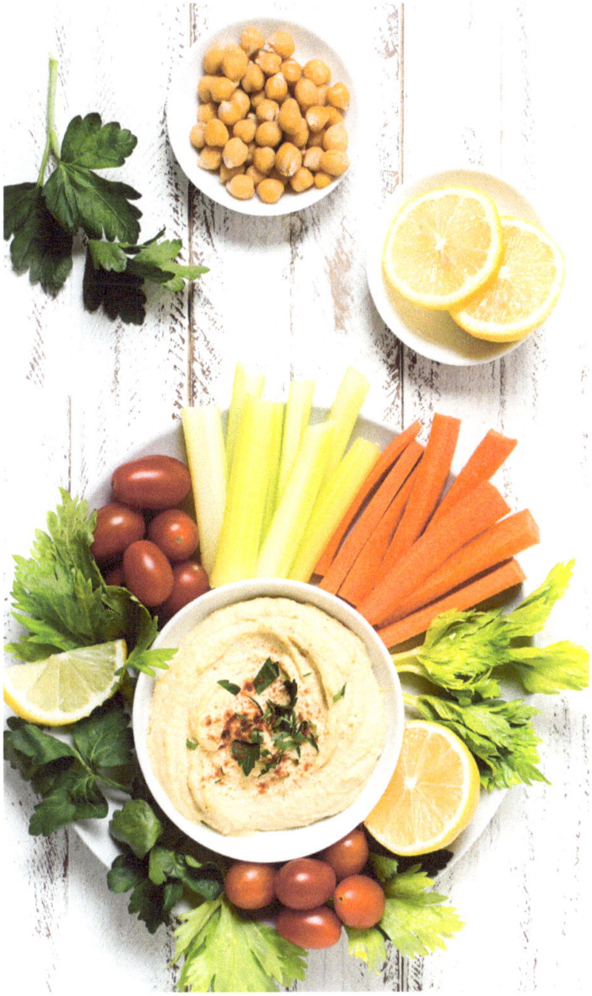

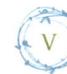

GF

Great Beginnings - Appetizers - Mezes - Snacks

Hummus with Veggies & Rolled Charcuterie

This is just one of those combos put together for a quick snack. I made some fresh hummus and thought I would combine it with some charcuterie for a tasty bite.

1 small ramekin of hummus
3 mini color peppers, sliced
4 slices of Italian salami
2 slices of your favorite cheese – "Graviera" is delicious
1 sprig of parsley
1 Kalamata olive, pitted

The full recipe for this tasty hummus is available in this cook book.

All you need to do is just cut up the peppers and assemble the rolls of cheese and salami and voila! It's an instant snack that is delicious and nutritious. You could make a bunch of those as an appetizer on a large platter when you have friends over.

Serves 1 person ***(All Seasons)***

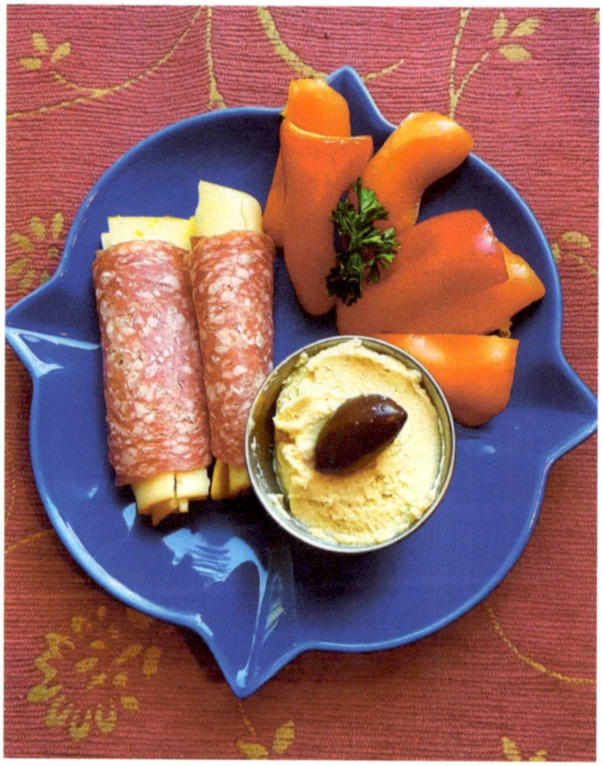

Pair with: Serve as a wholesome appetizer.

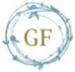

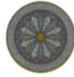

DF GF V

Greek Deviled Eggs

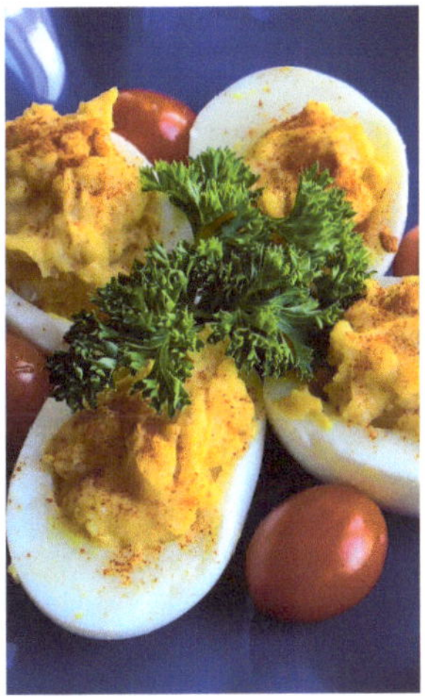

A quick and easy recipe that differs a little bit each time I make it depending on what is available in the fridge. Mayonnaise is not much to my liking, so I use a mayo substitute to bring this recipe together. Paprika, chopped roasted red peppers, relish and chopped celery are some other options I have added to this mix at times. The recipe below has more of a classic taste to it but if you love to cook, try different flavors for a unique experience. This is a quick appetizer to prepare and everyone seems to like it. Using farm fresh eggs enhances the taste even more.

- 6 farm fresh eggs
- ¼ cup Vegenaise
- 2 tsp. English type mustard
- ⅛ tsp. turmeric
- • Dash of paprika to top
- • Salt + pepper to taste

Boil eggs for about 6 mins and let cool. Peel and cut eggs in half, lengthwise. Scoop out egg yolk and put in small bowl. Arrange white part of eggs in a large flat platter. With a fork break down and mix egg yolks with Vegenaise, mustard, turmeric, salt and pepper. When mixture is well blended, fill the center of each egg enough to make a small heap. Sprinkle Paprika on top and serve.

Deviled eggs can be served by themselves as breakfast or an appetizer or you can use them as a topping in a salad.

P.S. You can add other ingredients to the mix as well depending on your preference. Some other ingredients that I have added at times are relish, capers and roasted red peppers.

Serves 5 people ***(All Seasons)***

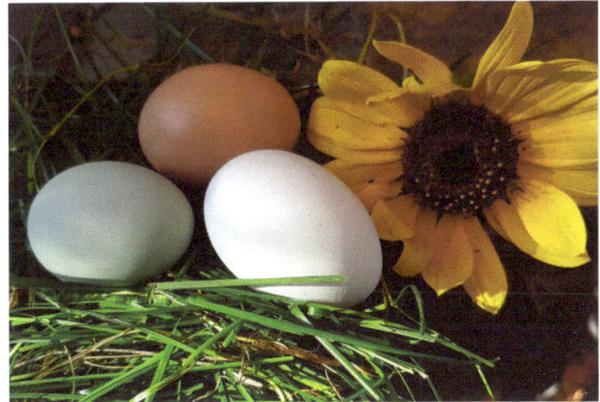

DF GF

Great Beginnings - Appetizers - Mezes - Snacks

Keftedakia - Small Baked Meat Balls

Κεφτεδάκια

One of my favorite childhood tastes. My mom often made Keftedakia when I was growing up, and I even remember sneaking up and eating some of the meat mixture while still raw. These meatballs are fluffy and delicious, although a bit more involved in preparation.

Originally this recipe calls for frying the Keftedakia in a pan of oil, but over the years we have adapted this recipe to be cooked in the oven. Since we are omitting the frying, we also do not need to roll the meatballs in flour. You can also make these bigger and serve them as an entrée with a nice vegetable side or salad.

- ½ lb. bread (GF if needed)
- 1 lb. organic ground beef
- 2 tbsp. olive oil
- 1 garlic clove, minced
- 3 eggs, beaten
- ¼ cup parsley, finely chopped
- 3 tbsp. mint, finely chopped (or 2 tbsp. dry mint)
- 3 tsp. oregano, finely chopped (or ½ tsp. dry oregano)
- ¼ tsp. grated nutmeg

This is a healthier version of the original Keftedakia, which is drenched in flour and fried.

Preheat oven to 375° F. Take a couple of thick slices of bread and soak in water, then squeeze out excess moisture. Remove crust and put in a large bowl. In the same bowl combine meat, olive oil, onions, garlic, eggs, herbs and spices. Knead all together until ingredients are well mixed.

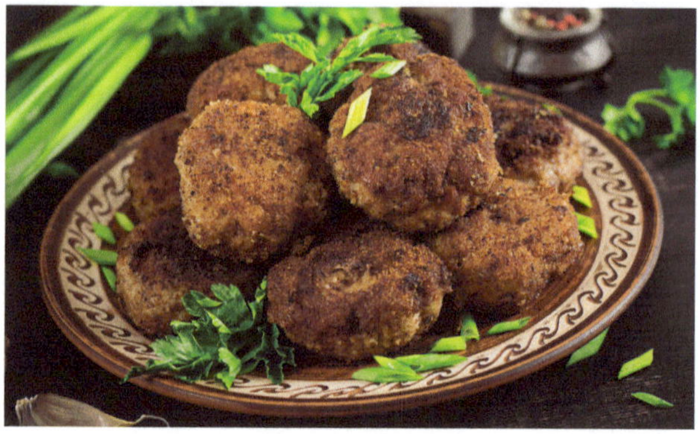

Shape small meatballs, about 1.5 inch in diameter and set aside on an ungreased oven tray about 2 inches apart. Bake for 15 minutes, turning the meatballs half way through with a fork or spatula. If you are making these bigger for a main entrée, make sure to allow more baking time so they can cook all the way through.

Remove tray from oven and let stand a few minutes. Keftedakia may be served hot or cold as finger food or alongside a side dish.

Serves 6 people ***(All Seasons)***

Pair with: Serve as an appetizer, or serve as a main dish with a crunchy cabbage salad.

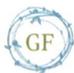

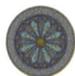

Melitzanosalata

Μελιτζανοσαλάτα

This is a classic Greek eggplant spread that has a very full and pungent flavor and can be very pulpy in texture. You often find this spread in tavernas, small restaurants in Greece, and it is good served with fried zucchini, a thick slice of village bread or try it with anything you might have on your plate. I have always enjoyed it even as a spread on top of meat or chicken.

- 2 medium eggplants
- 4 cloves of garlic, minced
- ½ cup olive oil
- 2 tbsp. white vinegar
- 1 tsp. sugar
  - Black olive, parsley or dill sprig for garnish
  - Olive oil for garnish
  - Salt to taste

Preheat oven to 375° F.

Wash eggplant and pat dry. Using a fork, make several holes in the eggplants and lay on an ungreased baking sheet. Bake whole for one hour or until the skin is shriveled and eggplant is nice and soft.

Take eggplant out of the oven, and while still hot, cut off stem and begin peeling the skin careful to not burn your fingers. Cut eggplant in half, lengthwise, and using a spoon remove as many of the seeds as you can without taking off the flesh of the eggplant. Using a fork, scrape the meat of the eggplant and put it in a glass bowl, add minced garlic and mix. Slowly drizzle and mix in olive oil and vinegar alternating while you are mixing. Add sugar and salt and continue to mix until well blended and you have reached your preferred consistency. Some like this spread pulpy and others prefer it smooth. Sprinkle some fresh olive oil on top. Serve warm.

Serves 8 people ***(Summer, Autumn)***

Pair with: Serve with cut up crunchy veggies or with pitta bread wedges.

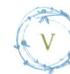

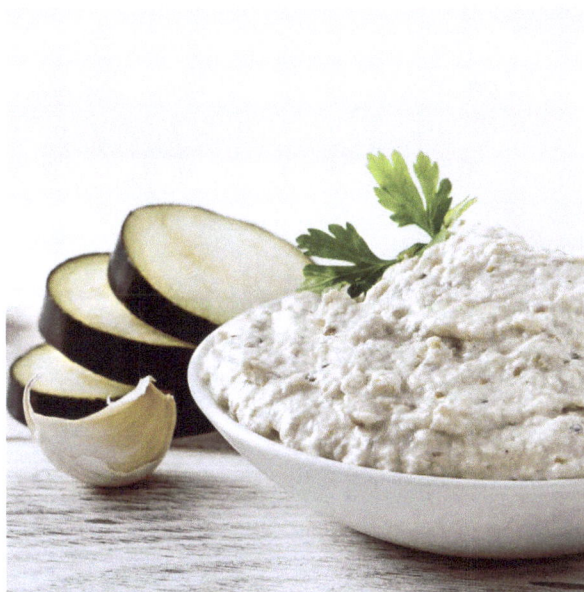

GF V

Kolokithokeftedes With Tzatziki Sauce

Κολοκυθοκεφτέδες με τζατζίκι

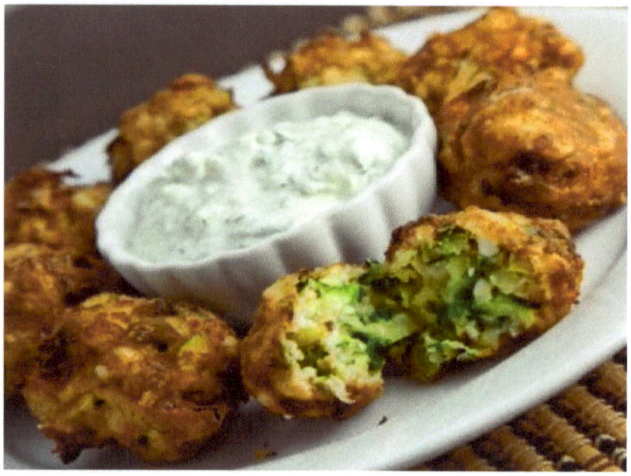

Kolokithokeftedes is Greek zucchini fritters with yoghurt sauce... There is something about the smooth soft taste of cooked zucchini that brings back fond memories in the kitchen. I can still see my mom in her apron covered in flour preparing these delicious fritters with zucchini and feta cheese. It makes my mouth water even as we speak. One of the problems of writing this cookbook over time is that writing out all these tasty recipes has made me hungry all the time!

This recipe is a leftover effect from making "Stuffed Zucchini" or "Kolokythakia Yemista". In the process of making the stuffed zucchini you remove the core (the insides) of the vegetable and fill it with rice, spices and herbs. The leftover "flesh" from the zucchini can be then chopped up and used to make the fritters.

For Fritters:

- 3 cups packed, grated zucchini (from about 6 large zucchini)
- 6 tbsps. fresh dill, chopped
- 1 bunch (about 8) scallions, white and light green parts finely chopped
- ½ tsp. nutmeg
- 1 ½ cups crumbled feta
- 4 large eggs, lightly beaten
- 1 cup flour (plus more if needed) (use gluten free flower mix for GF version)
- • Salt + pepper to taste
- 4 tbsps. olive oil or more for frying

For Tzatziki:

- 2 cups Greek strained yogurt
- 1 clove of garlic, minced
- ½ cup grated, peeled cucumber
- 1 tsp. lemon juice
- 1 tbsp. Greek olive oil
- • Salt + pepper to taste

For the Fritters: Spread out grated zucchini in a large colander, sprinkle with salt and let sit for at least 30 min-

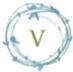

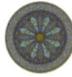

GF V

Kolokithokeftedes with Tzatziki Sauce

Κολοκυθοκεφτέδες με τζατζίκι

utes to release most of its liquid. Squeeze out any excess moisture with your hands and in a large bowl mix with dill, scallions, nutmeg, and feta and combine well. Stir in eggs and season with salt and pepper. Mix in flour until it forms a dense dough and you can form patties about 3-4 inches big.

Heat olive oil in a large skillet over medium high heat. Add each patty to the hot frying pan and cook until crisp, turning the patties over half way, about 3 minutes on each side depending on the thickness of your patty.

Fry patties until golden brown on both sides and cooked through but still moist. Prepare a plate lined with paper towels to absorb the oil from the fritters. Serve hot with tzatziki alongside.

Tzatziki: Grate cucumber and let sit for a while. Then squeeze excess moisture from the batch. In a small bowl, mix yogurt, minced garlic, cucumber and lemon juice. Stir in olive oil. Add salt and pepper to taste and keep in fridge until fritters are ready.

Serves 4 people (8 fritters) ***(Late Summer)***

Pair with: Serve as an appetizer, or serve as a side dish with steaks and salad.

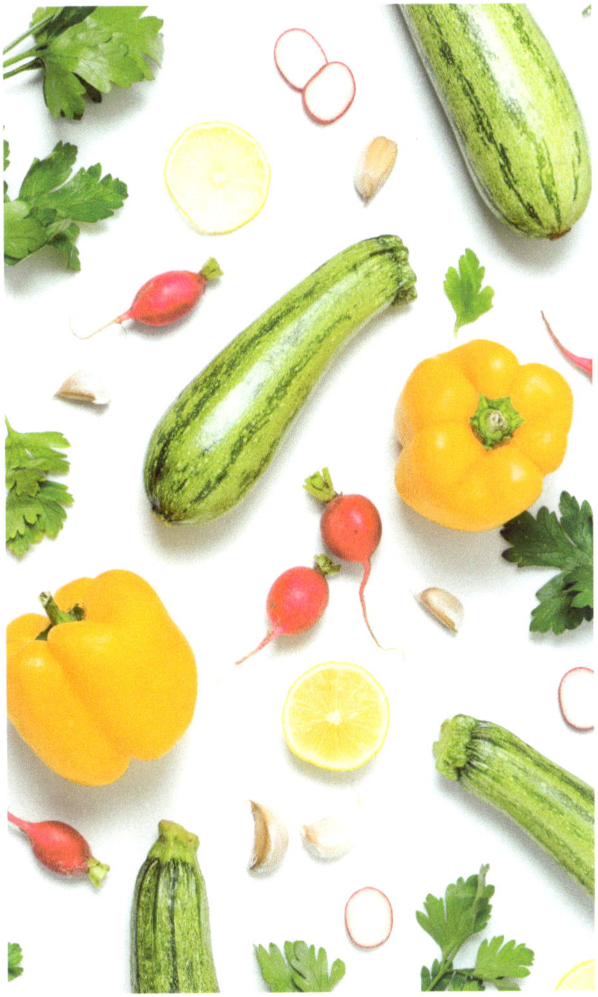

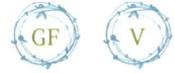

V

Pitta Bread, Greek Style

Πίττα

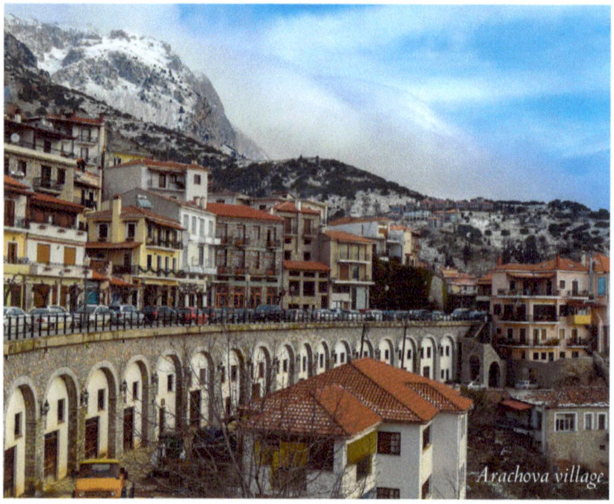

Arachova village

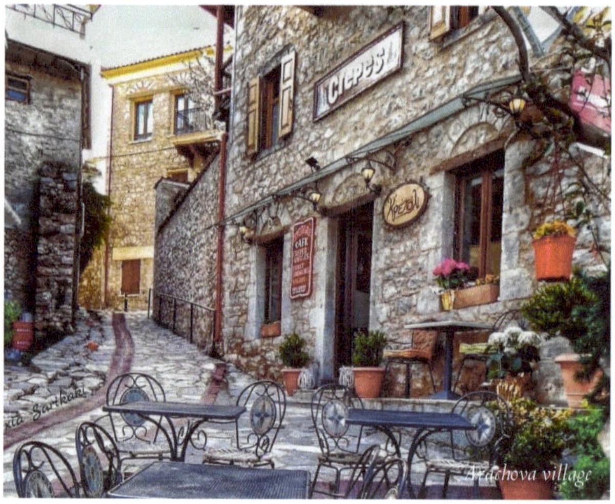

Arachova village

Pitta is a staple in Greece, right alongside some fresh home cooked bread. This is an easy recipe but an elaborate process. It can be used as an accompaniment to many Mediterranean dishes. A classic pitta recipe can be served alongside any meal, either as an accompaniment or to fill with your favorites and make a type of rolled sandwich.

One of the most popular Greek dishes, Souvlaki, is small pieces of grilled pork wrapped in a pitta and filled with tomatoes, onions and tzatziki sauce.

When I was a teenager, we used to get up early in the morning to catch the 5:00 am bus to the mountains and go skiing. At lunch time we would always stop at this tiny restaurant, a hole in the wall, literally, at the foot of Mt. Parnassós. They served a mean souvlaki and made the best pitta in the village of Arachova.

- 2 envelopes active dry yeast
- 1 tsp. sugar
- 2 cups warm water
- 6-7 cups all-purpose flour
- 2 tsp. salt
- 5 tsp. butter, melted cornmeal

Dissolve yeast and sugar in 1 cup of warm water, and cover with a clean towel to keep warm. Let it stand in

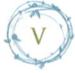

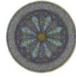

Pitta Bread, Greek Style

Πίττα

a warm place for about 15 minutes until it has formed bubbles.

In a large bowl combine flour and salt. Form a well in the center of the bowl and add remaining 1 cup of warm water, melted butter and bubbly yeast and start mixing with a wooden spoon until you have a sticky dough. Take a little bit of the flour and sprinkle on a clean surface where you can start kneading the dough. Continue kneading until you have a silky mixture, adding a little bit of flour during the process as you go. If batter sticks to your fingers, add a bit more flour and rub off your hands continuing to knead.

Once you have the silky dough ready, form a large ball and place in an oiled covered bowl for about 1 ½ hours until it has doubled in size. Take the dough and punch it down again and then let it rest for another 20 minutes.

Prepare a couple of baking sheets by sprinkling cornmeal on top. Take the dough and divide into half, and half again and again until you have 10-12 small balls. Roll out each ball into an 8 inch circle, place in prepared pan about an inch away from each other. Cover again with a towel and place in a warm place for 30 minutes, allowing the dough to rest.

Meanwhile, preheat the oven to 500 F. After 30 minutes take the first tray and place it in lower rack in oven and bake until each circle forms a bubble, about 4-5 minutes. Then move tray to the middle rack for another 5 minutes. Repeat with the second tray. Take out of the oven and allow pitta to cool a little before serving.

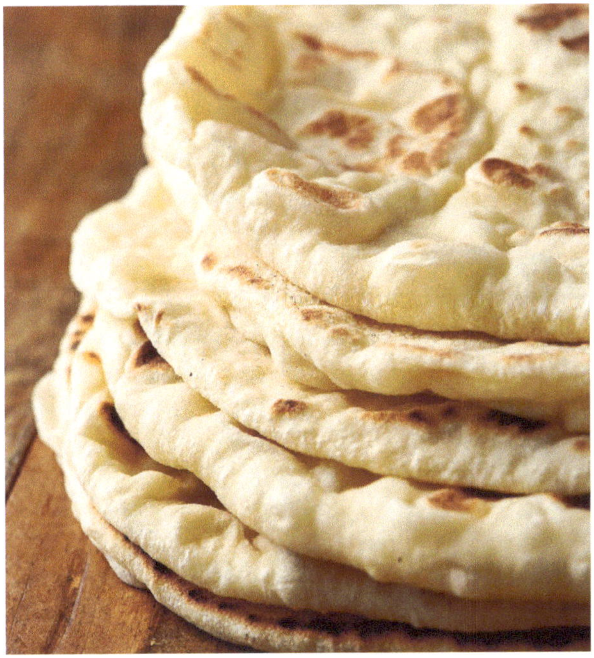

You may serve pitta hot or cold and since it is such an elaborate process you can also put some in the freezer for future use.

Serves 10 people ***(Year round)***

Pair with: serve with any dish on the side or as a sandwich wrap

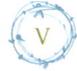

DF GF

Great Beginnings - Appetizers - Mezes - Snacks

Grilled Octopus

Χταπόδι στη σχάρα

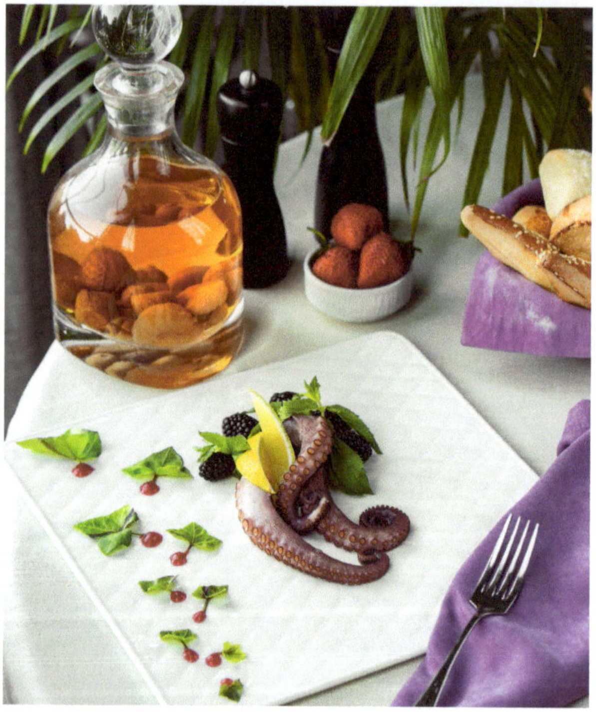

While strolling in the islands of Greece, you will often come across the view of freshly caught octopus laid out to dry in the sun before being prepared for a meal. Prior to that the fishermen will literally beat and wash the octopus on the rocks until it froths to make it soft and easy to eat. We used to go spearfishing for octopus when I was young and when my dad would catch one, he would chase us in the sea with the octopus waving its limbs in the water and sometimes he would catch us, wrapping their tentacles around us!

Usually the octopi were not too large and removing the suckers was easy, but to this day I remember the plopping sound they made as we would pull them off our skin and the red dots it would leave for a while!

We enjoy octopus either grilled or cooked in a pot with a vinegar sauce. This recipe is a quick appetizer with a very unique taste. Octopus loses a lot of its volume during cooking, so be prepared to have about half of what you start with.

- 1 large fresh octopus (2-3 lbs.)
- ½ cup water or red wine if needed
- 1 bay leaf
- ½ cup olive oil
- 2 tbsps. red wine vinegar
- ½ tsp. dry crushed Greek oregano
  - Salt + pepper to taste

To Serve:

- 1 tbsp. olive oil
- ½ tsp. dry oregano
- 1 lemon to squeeze over grilled octopus

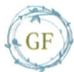

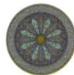

GF DF

Grilled Octopus

Χταπόδι στη σχάρα

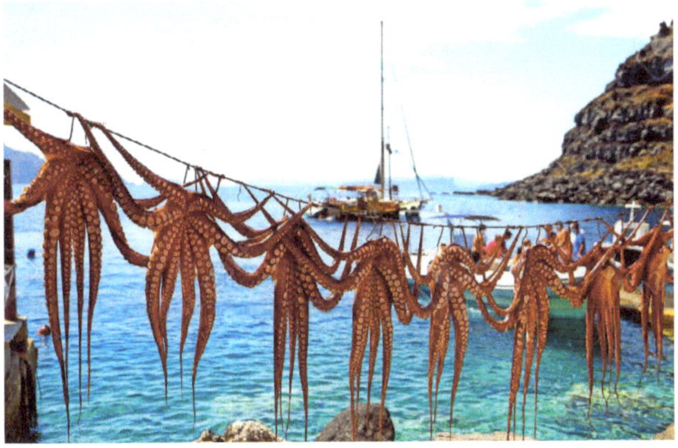

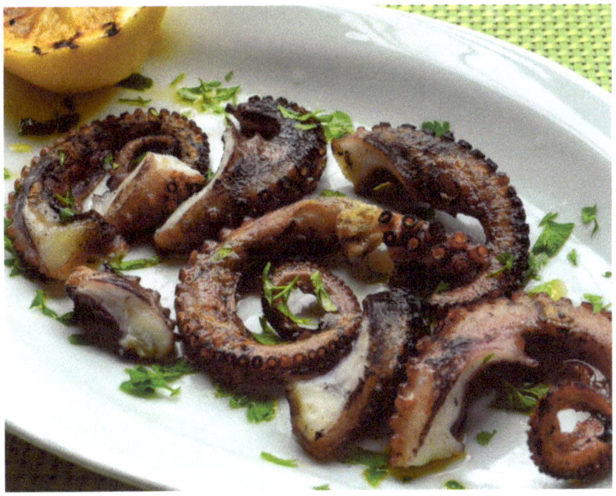

Rinse your octopus well under running water and then place in a large enough pot over high heat and cover allowing about 10 minutes for the liquid to be released from the octopus. If your octopus is frozen, allow it to thaw in a bowl in the fridge completely before rinsing under cold water. Lower the heat to low and braise octopus for about an hour depending on its size.

If your liquid evaporates during this process, you may add some water or red wine to continue. This will make the octopus easy to grill and eat. You may add some herbs into the pot such as a bay leaf, and some Greeks swear by adding the cork of a red wine into the braising pot to help the process along. I have not tried this, but if you do, let me know how it turns out.

Use a fork to discern the tenderness of the octopus and if it is soft enough, remove from the pot and into a bowl.

Add some olive oil, red wine vinegar, fresh oregano, salt and pepper and let stand until the octopus has reached room temperature. Cover and let stand in the fridge overnight to marinade.

Prepare your grill, drain the dressing of the octopus and lay on a hot fire to sear. This only takes a few minutes, as the octopus is already cooked for the most part. To serve, remove from the grill onto a cutting board and either cut in pieces or slices. Cover with a bit of olive oil, sprinkle a bit dry oregano and drizzle some lemon juice on top and enjoy.

Serves 6 people ***(Summer, Fall)***

Pair with: Serve as an appetizer

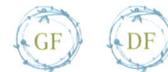

DF GF V *Great Beginnings - Appetizers - Mezes - Snacks*

Rice Flour Cauliflower

Κουνουπίδι στον φούρνο

This lightly breaded and baked recipe makes a delicious appetizer, and is great topped with some spicy sauce or yoghurt sauce. Vegetarian appetizers are some of my favorite foods. To this day baked cauliflower, roasted Brussel sprouts, crunchy kale and spicy eggplant are foods that we indulge in often. When our children where young and I would bake kale chips, the kids from around the neighborhood would come enjoy them. They could smell it all the way from their house and stop by for a snack. Just like cauliflower, kale chips are not only delicious and crunchy but they are also filled with nutrition.

1 large cauliflower head
2 - 3 medium eggs, beaten (depending on the size of the cauliflower)
¼ cup all-purpose or GF flour, rice is a great light option
1 tsp. paprika
- Salt + Pepper
4 tbsp. olive oil
½ cup parmesan cheese to sprinkle on top (optional)

Preheat oven to 400° F.

Wash cauliflower head and cut off the big stem, separating flowerets into small pieces. In a separate large bowl beat 2-3 eggs and add cauliflower to it and toss until all flowerets are well covered. Mix flour with spices and generously sprinkle over flowerets and continuously toss until they are all well covered.

Loosely lay out cauliflower in a large shallow and greased oven pan and spray with olive oil to set the flour. Bake in oven for 25 minutes, until golden brown on top. Remove from oven and serve immediately.

Serves 6 people ***(Autumn, Winter, Spring)***

Pair with: Serve as an appetizer

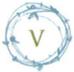

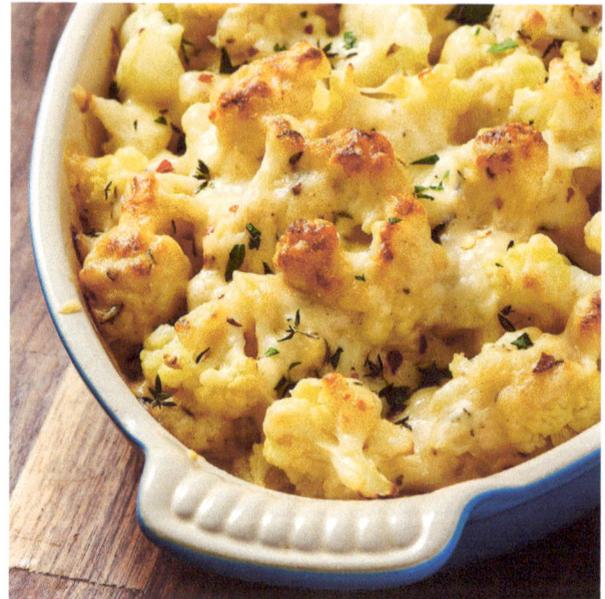

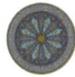

GF V

Saganaki - A Fried Cheese Dish

Σαγανάκι

A great side dish that is usually served as an appetizer and often enjoyed with an Ouzo; a Greek anise drink. You might often see this dish at a restaurant arrive in flames as a flambé. As they set it on the table, they put the flames out by squeezing some fresh lemon juice on it. Crunchy on the outside and gooey warm on the inside it is a delectable dish that will leave you craving more.

- ½ lb. kefalotyri, halloumi or any hard and salty yellow cheese. Can also be made with feta cheese.
- ¼ cup all-purpose or GF flour
- 4 tbsp. olive oil
- 1 lemon, juiced

Cut cheese into 3 inch long pieces about ½ inch thick. In Greece it is usually cut in triangles or long pieces.

Lightly wet cheese with water and gently pat try so it becomes sticky. Cover with flour and shake off excess. Most of these cheeses are pretty salty so you do not need to add any salt.

Heat the olive oil in a heavy skillet in medium fire, and when hot, add the dredged cheese into the pan and cook for about 3 minutes on each side. Remove cheese, sprinkle lemon juice and serve warm.

Serves 6 people ***(All Seasons)***

Pair with: Serve as an appetizer

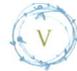

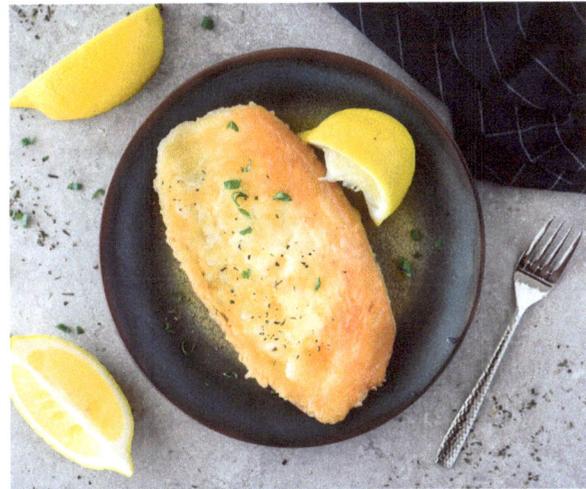

GF V

Tzatziki Dip

Τζατζίκι

A sauce to dip just about everything in it, if you are fond of yoghurt & garlic.

2 cups Greek strained yoghurt

2 cloves of garlic, minced (double if you prefer)

½ cup grated, cucumber

1 ½ tbsps. finely chopped dill or mint (your preference)

1 ½ tbsps. red wine vinegar or 1 teaspoon lemon juice

1 tbsp. Greek olive oil

- Salt to taste

Tzatziki: Grate cucumber and let sit for a while (at least an hour or so). Then squeeze excess moisture from the batch by either squeezing out small batches between your hands or pushing it through a sieve. In a small bowl, mix yoghurt, minced garlic, herbs, cucumber and vinegar/lemon juice. Stir in olive oil. Add salt to taste and keep in the fridge until ready to eat. Garnishing with olives and parsley makes a nice presentation.

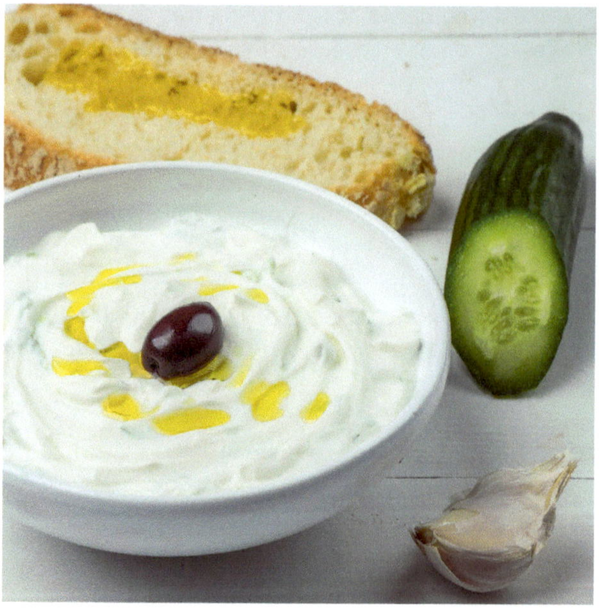

Serves 8 people ***(Summer, Autumn)***

Pair with: Cut up crunchy veggies - carrots, celery, jicama root - or serve with pitta bread wedges. Also great with vegetable fritters, or served next to meat dishes.

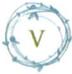

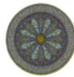

GF DF

Tuna Salad Sandwich

This is such an easy lunch or snack option that we often prepare it in our kitchen. A good source of protein and veggies while at the same time it leaves you satisfied and content. Since we are not big on mayo, we substitute an egg free version for this recipe but you can use either. Not only can you serve it on bread as a sandwich, but you can also make mini appetizers on crackers or serve it on a bed of lettuce.

It is a healthy source of protein and I love to combine it with freshly cut veggies on the side, such as carrot and celery wedges, cherry tomatoes and lettuce leaves.

- 2 cups tuna fish packed in water or olive oil
- 1 cup shredded carrots
- ½ cup finely chopped celery
- ½ cup finely chopped red onion
- ¼ cup finely chopped dill pickles or relish
- ¼ cup finely chopped fresh parsley (optional)
- 1 cup mayonnaise or other egg/soy free alternative
- 1 tbsp. Greek olive oil
- ½ tsp. red wine vinegar
- • Salt + Pepper to taste

Place tuna in a large bowl to mix with remaining ingredients.

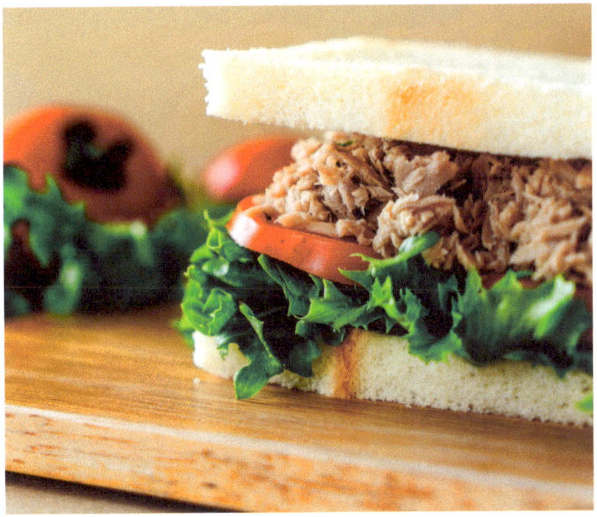

Add carrots, celery, onion, dill and parsley and mix well. In a separate small bowl combine mayonnaise with olive oil and mix until well incorporated.

Add vinegar, salt and pepper and blend. Add mayonnaise mixture to tuna bowl and mix well.

Serve your favorite way.

Serves 8 people
(Summer, Autumn)

Pair with: Cut up crunchy veggies - carrots, celery, jicama root - or serve as a sandwich on wheat or gluten free bread slices.

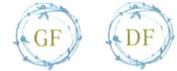

3

Warm and Soothing Soups

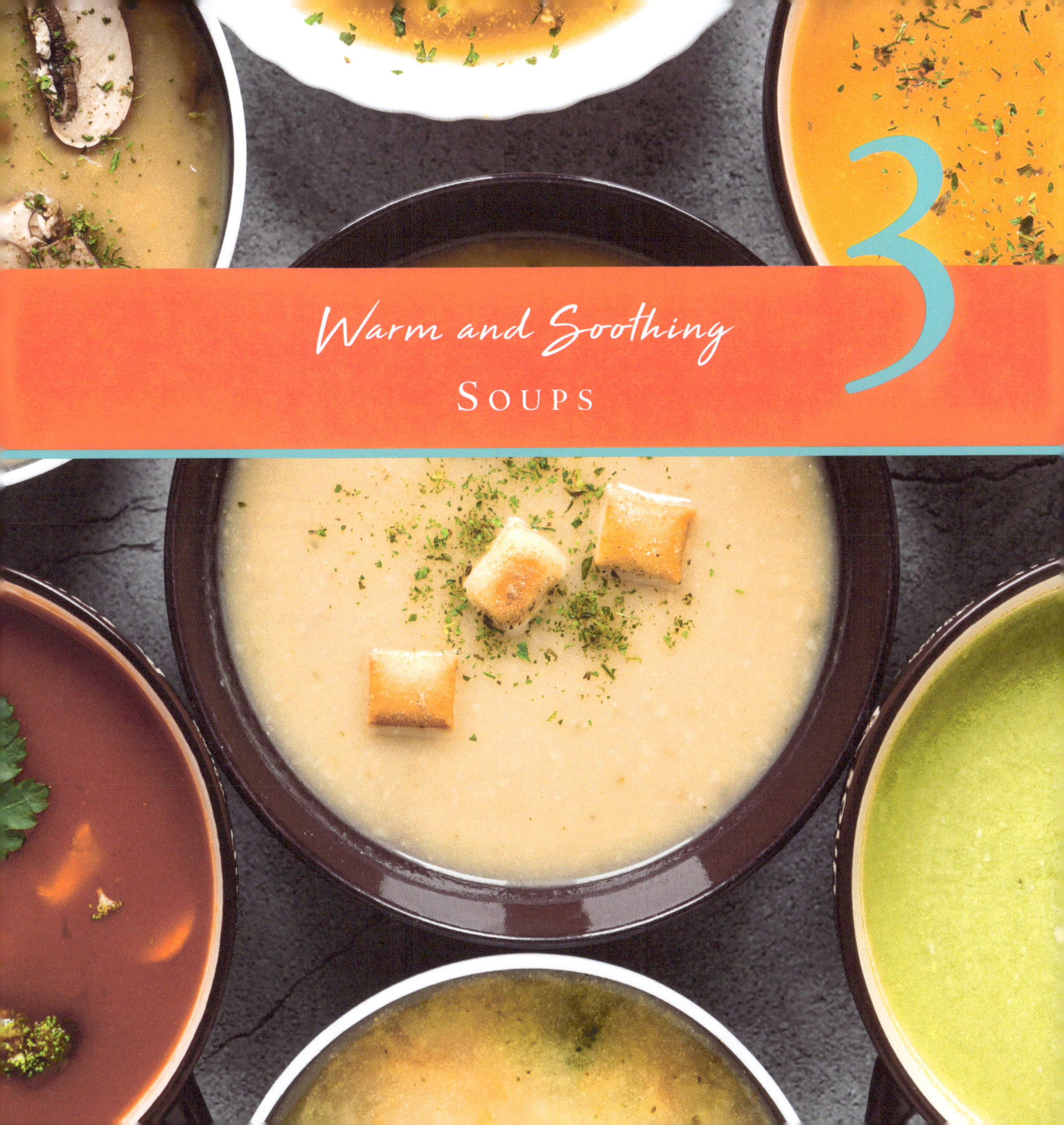

DF GF V

Carrot Ginger soup

Σούπα καρότο

A simple but soothing cold weather soup that is filling and healing. Both carrots and ginger have lots of vitamins and immune boosting ingredients. You can adjust the texture of this soup by blending a little or a lot once it is cooked. My preference is blending it really smooth to where it becomes a velvety experience in your mouth.

4 tbsp. olive oil

10 large carrots, cleaned and cut in rounds

1 ½ cups grated yellow onion

4 cups organic vegetable broth

1 cup of water

2 tbsp. grated ginger

¼ cup fresh finely chopped chives

- Salt + Pepper to taste
- Dollop of half & half in serving bowl (omit for DF)

In a large pot sauté the onions and carrots on a medium fire for about 8 minutes until they are slightly soft but not browned. Add broth, water, ginger, salt and pepper and bring to boil. Cook on medium heat for about 10 more minutes.

Transfer some of the soup into your blender, making sure to fill only about 2/3, as the steam and heat will make it harder to keep covered and it tends to spill out of a full container. Blend mixture to your desired texture and empty in a serving dish. Repeat with remaining soup until it is all done.

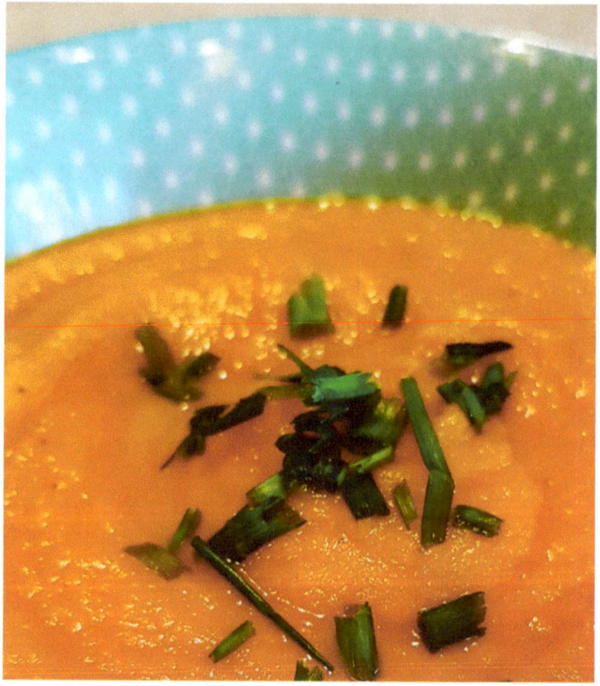

Add chives as a garnish and serve with a piece of toasted bread or pitta bread on the side.

Serves 6 people *(Autumn, Winter)*

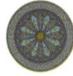

DF GF V

Tomato Soup

Ντοματόσουπα

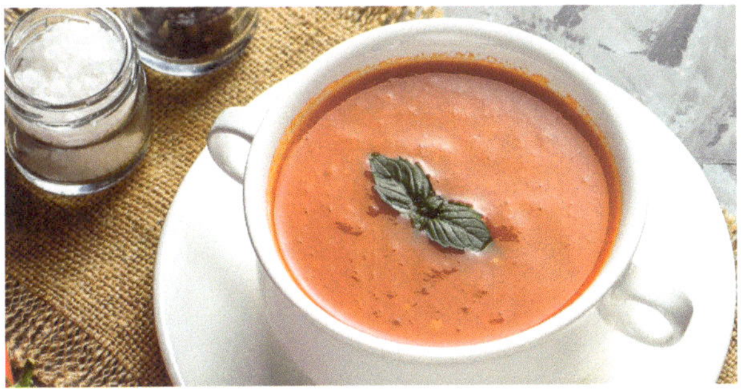

A smooth and silky tomato soup is one of my fondest memories from my childhood. After washing the tomatoes, I cut them in half and then gently grate the flesh into a bowl until only the skin is left. I find this is an easy way of harvesting most of the tomato flesh while discarding the skin and core. This year our tomato harvest was so abundant that we had the opportunity to enjoy a delicious tomato soup throughout autumn.

You will notice that the option of adding Trahana is available instead of rice. Trahana is an ancient dried food ingredient, based on a fermented mixture of grain and yoghurt or milk. It is found in the cuisines of Southeast Europe and the Middle East. It has a texture of coarse, uneven crumbs, and it is usually made into a thick soup with water, stock, or milk. In Greece it is readily available and I usually bring a few bags back with me when we travel. In the US you might be able to find it in International and Mediterranean markets or order it online. If you are concerned about allergies this is not a gluten or dairy free food.

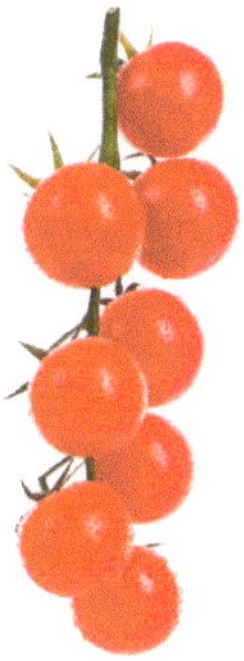

- 3 tbsps. olive oil
- 1 medium Vidalia onion, finely chopped
- 6 lbs. plum large tomatoes peeled & chopped
- 10 cups of water
- 1 garlic glove, minced
- 1 tsp. raw sugar
- 1 tbsp. sea salt
- Fresh ground pepper to taste
- ½ cup long grain rice, or bulgur or trahana
- ¼ cup fresh chopped parsley or
- 1 tsp. dry parsley
- 2 tbsp. red wine vinegar

In a large pot add olive oil and onions and sauté until they are translucent, about 4 minutes over medium heat. Add fresh grated tomatoes, water, minced garlic, sugar, salt and pepper and simmer covered for about 30 minutes.

Remove the cover and add the rice, bulgur or trahana into the pot. Mix well and if needed add more water, as the rice will be absorbing a lot of it as it cooks. Mix again, raise fire to medium high and bring to a gentle boil, then cover pot, bring fire to low and simmer for another 20 minutes. Remove cover and add parsley and vinegar and mix once more. Let it sit for about five minutes before serving.

Serves 6 people ***(Autumn, Winter)***

Pair with: This dish is paired well with a green salad, some fresh baked bread and a full bodied red wine.

DF GF

Warm and Soothing - Soups

Chicken Soup – Greek Style

Κοτόσουπα Αυγολέμονο

This soup is a go to for a cold night or anytime someone in the family is not feeling well. Whether it is the combination of ingredients or the gesture of someone making you soup to help you feel better, it always brings a soothing feeling and gentle warmth. This soup has been one of my favorites since I was a child, and it is our family's favorite as well to this day. The cloves in the onion adds a lot of goodness to boost the immune system and the chicken bone broth is also very strengthening. Free range chickens, raised with organic feed and without antibiotics are always a plus. Since I do not always have 2-3 hours to spare to slow cook the chicken, I often make it in the pressure cooker and it is just as good.

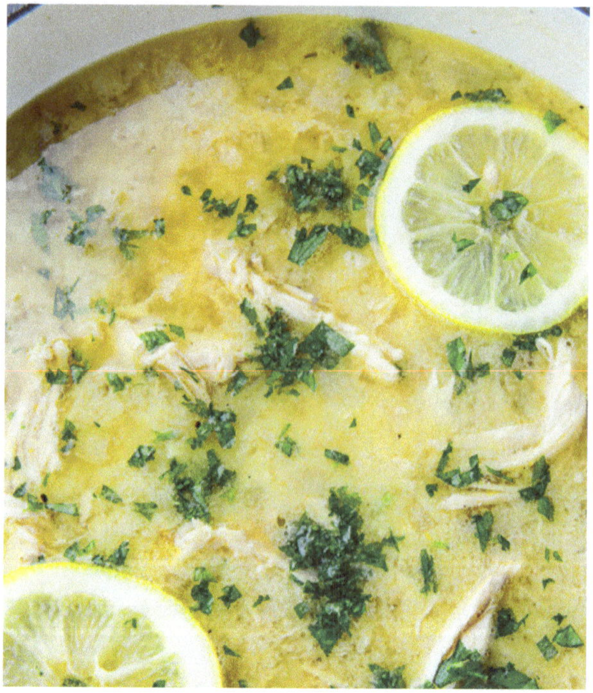

- 1 medium to large roasting chicken (4 - 5lbs.)
- 1 large yellow onion, unpeeled and studded with 4 cloves (just remove any dirty outer layers)
- 2 ½ quarts water
- Salt + Pepper to taste
- 1 cup long grain rice (your preference)
- 2-3 eggs at room temperature
- 2 large lemons, juiced
  - Additional freshly ground black pepper to season bowl

Wash and dry chicken inside out before cooking. In a large pot (or large pressure cooker) bring chicken, studded onion, and water to a slow boil. In the beginning, as the pot begins to boil, skim off any foam that forms on the top until it stops foaming. Add salt and pepper and simmer covered for 2 ½ to 3 hours. If you are using a pressure cooker, put the lid on the pot, seal pressure cooker, and bring up to pressure. Cook 3 minutes for each pound. For example, if your chicken weighs 4 lbs., cook under pressure for 12 minutes.

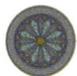

GF DF

Chicken Soup – Greek Style

Κοτόσουπα Αυγολέμονο

When the chicken is done it will be so soft that the meat will fall off the bone.

Remove chicken and onion from the pot onto a large tray to cool. I like to use a baking tray to spread out the chicken while I debone it, separate and chop smaller pieces for the soup. If using a pressure cooker make sure to follow the instructions for your pot and release pressure before removing the lid.

While chicken is cooling off, add rice to the pot and simmer for 15 minutes. Meanwhile, debone chicken and cut into small pieces to your liking. Add the chicken to the pot with the rice and simmer ajar, another 5 minutes. You might need to add more water to the pot as it cooks down, and to achieve your preferred consistency.

While the soup is cooking, gather your lemon juice and eggs to make the avgolemono sauce. In a medium bowl beat together eggs until they are well blended and then slowly add in lemon juice while still beating the mixture.

The goal is to mix slowly so that eggs and lemon combine into a smooth and frothy mixture.

Once that is done, very slowly, drizzle 4 to 5 ladles of soup broth into the egg mixture, continuing to whisk vigorously so the eggs will not curdle.

Remove the pot from the fire and pour the sauce mixture slowly back into the pot, stirring gently with a wooden spoon.

Serve while warm and season with some fresh cracked pepper on top of each bowl. Black pepper is also very good for our immune system and helps the body recover its strength.

Serves 8 people ***(Autumn, Winter)***

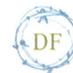

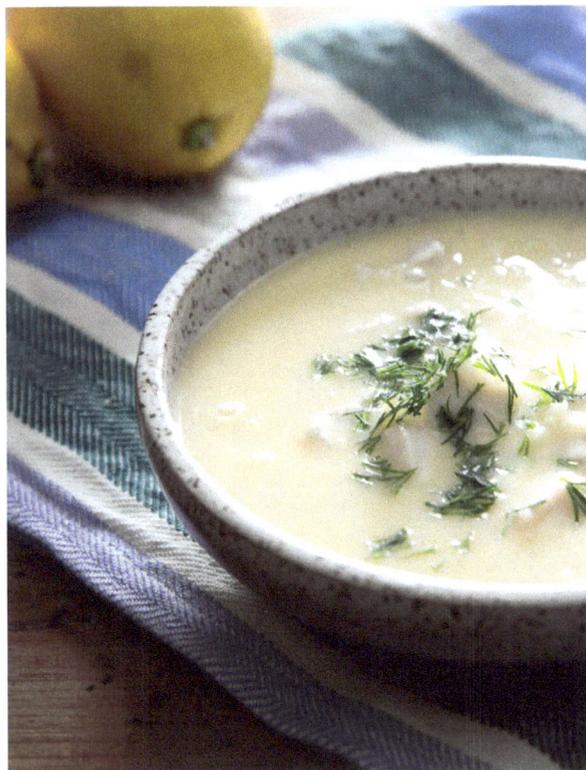

DF GF V

Fakes - Lentil Soup With A German Inspiration

Φακές

This is more or less my mother's recipe, who spent a large part of her young life in Germany. Hence, a lot of her cooking was influenced by the culture of that country and so many of the recipes I grew up with also had that German inspiration.

When I was growing up, I was not particularly fond of lentils but fast forward a few years and this recipe became one of my favorite winter meals.

To this day, it is often enjoyed by our family especially since it is a speedy and tasty meal for a cold evening. The addition of carrots make it a bit sweet and the sausage adds depth and texture to the flavor. If you prefer the vegetarian option, you may omit the sausages and it is still just as delicious and filling.

- 2 cups green lentils
- ¼ cup olive oil
- 2 large onions, chopped coarsely
- 4 large carrots, cut in chunks
- 2 garlic gloves, minced
- 8 cups water
- ¼ cup fresh parsley, finely chopped
- 1 large bay leaf
- 1 small, dry, red chili pepper, whole (optional)
- 4 Frankfurt sausages, sliced thick (optional)
  - Salt + Pepper to taste
- 2 tbsps. red wine vinegar

A pressure cooker is my preferred way of cooking my lentils, but if you do not own one, then a large deep pot will do. In your pot heat up the olive oil and sauté the onions until translucent. Add carrots and sauté for few more minutes and then add garlic, stirring constantly with a wooden spoon.

Add dry lentils and mix and sauté for about three more minutes before adding the water. Throw in the bay leaf, an entire hot pepper, salt, pepper, water and seal the pressure cooker, if you are using one. Check your pressure cooker manual as different sized pots will have different cooking times.

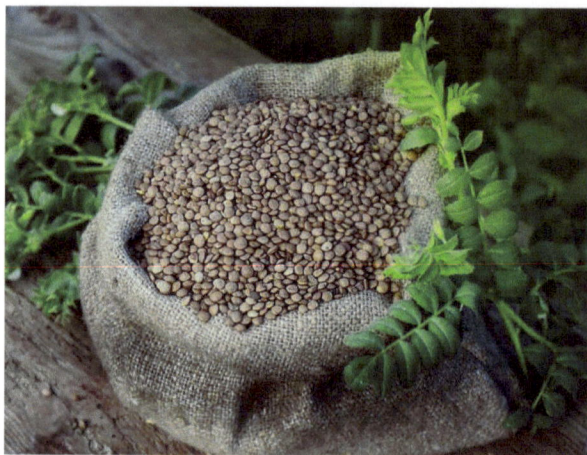

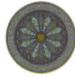

Fakes - Lentil Soup With A German Inspiration

Φακές

I find that 6 minutes is all it takes once the pressure cooker has reached its steaming zenith. When the time has elapsed, remove the cooker from the fire and allow it to slowly lose all its steam before opening up the pot. Add the cut up sausages and bring the pot back to a boil. Remove from fire and let it rest for about 5 minutes. Then add the red wine vinegar by gently mixing it into the soup.

If you are cooking in a normal pot, cover lentils, bring to a boil, then reduce heat to low and simmer for about 1 to 1 ½ hours until lentils are done and carrots are tender. If you like your soups more liquid add some water during cooking. About 5 minutes before lentils are ready, add the chopped sausage sand bring back to a boil. Cook for another 2 minutes then remove pot from heat and let it rest for a few minutes. Add red wine vinegar gently mixing it in and serve.

We like a lot of vinegar in our soup, but start off with a little bit until you find your preferred amount.

You do not want to overcook your lentils to where they become a soft mass, but instead just soft enough while the lentils still keep their shape. Make sure to check your pot often so you can taste the progress of your soup.

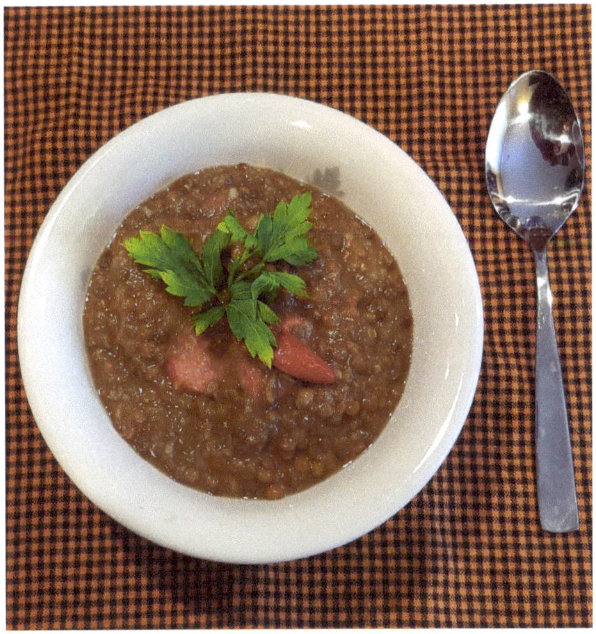

Serves 6 people ***(Autumn, Winter, Spring)***

Pair with: This dish is very filling and is served by itself in Greece, perhaps with a hearty slice of warm seeded bread. For a vegetarian option simply omit the sausage.

DF GF V

Fassolatha - Baby Lima Bean Soup

Φασολάδα

Olympus mountain

This is one of my very favorite soups for winter time! It reminds me of when I was a young adult and we used to go up to Mount Olympus for a winter excursion. Mount Olympus is the highest mountain in Greece, located in the Olympus Range on the border between Thessalia and Macedonia. It's highest peak rises to 2,917 meters or 9,570 feet.

If you are not familiar with this mountain, Olympus is one of the most prominent mountains in Greece, also the home of the twelve Greek Gods and the site of the throne of Zeus in Greek mythology. On our way down from the mountain, we would stop at the shelter where they served the best Fassolatha soup, especially after a cold and wintery day on the slopes. It is a smooth and soothing soup, and it might become your favorite just like mine.

Beans are a food rich in fiber, high in protein, iron and vitamin B. Because of this, Fassolada soup, just like the Greek chicken soup, is perfect for the winter flu! With the help of its hefty dose of olive oil present in this recipe, this becomes one of the healthier recipes which the heart-healthy Mediterranean diet is praised for.

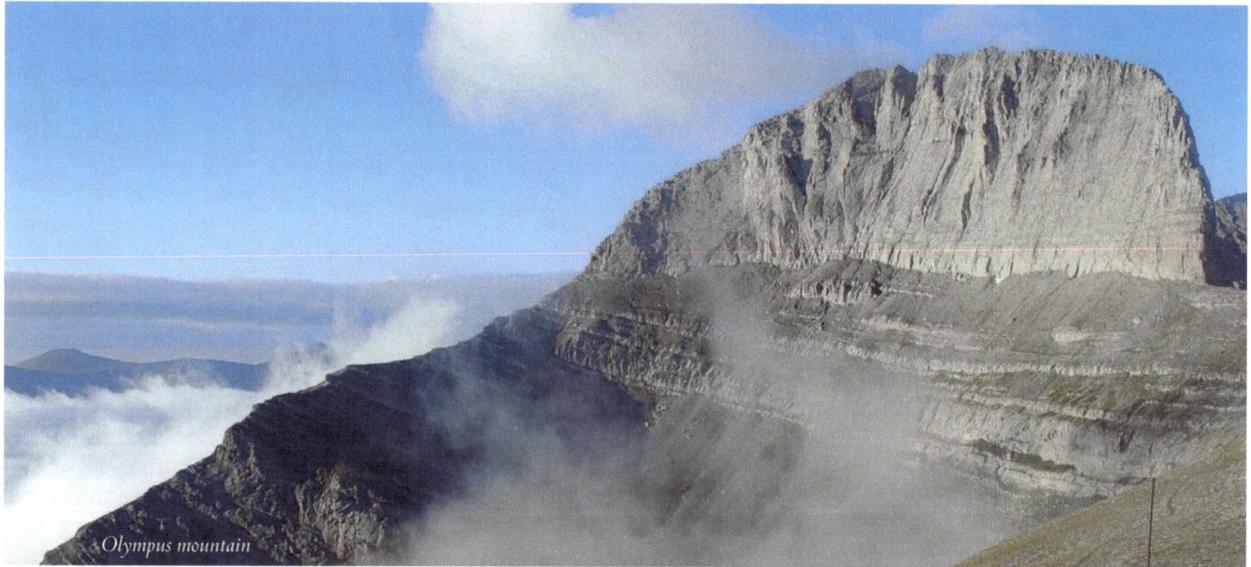

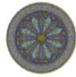

DF GF V

Fassolatha - Baby Lima Bean Soup

Φασολάδα

- ¼ cup olive oil
- 2 onions, diced
- 3 carrots, sliced thick
- 2 celery sticks with leaves, sliced thick
- 12 cups of water
- 1 cup lima beans or "yiyandes" beans (from Greece) rinsed & soaked for at least 8 hours or overnight.
- 8 soft, plum tomatoes, peeled and chopped
  - Salt + Pepper to taste
- 1 fresh strained juice of one lemon

In Greece there are at least a couple of white type beans, small and large, that are often used in our recipes. One of them called "yiyandes" (giant) are used often in baked dishes and they are like navy beans but 4 times as big. The smaller ones are often used for soups or other baked vegetarian dishes. While it is really hard to find those beans where we are, lima beans make just as delicious of a soup.

After soaking the beans overnight, take a large soup pot and fill with water and olive oil and bring to boil. Meanwhile, sauté onions, carrots and celery for about five minutes until they soften. Stir vegetables into pot with water and add beans, tomatoes, salt and pepper and bring to a rolling boil for a couple of minutes. Lower heat and simmer beans for about 2 hours. Add more water, if necessary, during cooking and bring back to a boil then lower heat. It might be closer to 2 ½ hours before the beans are tender and the soup is ready. Turn off the heat and pour in lemon juice in the end. Serve warm and enjoy.

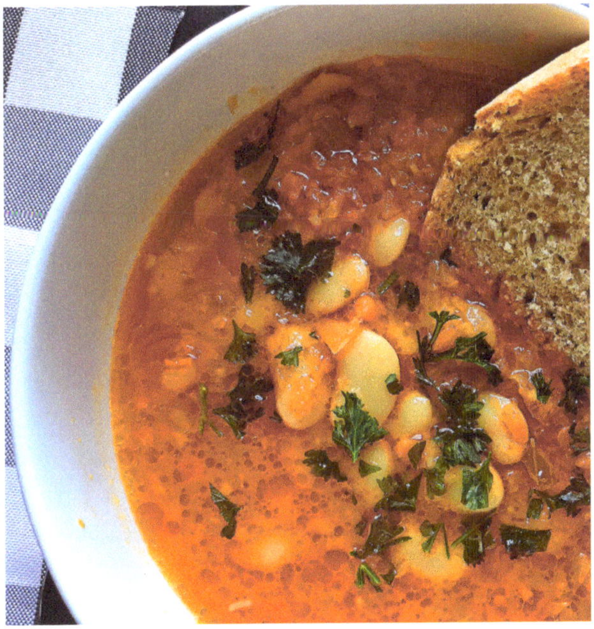

Serves 6 people ***(Autumn, Winter)***

Pair with: In Greece we enjoy this soup by itself or with a thick slice of bread to dip in.

Fide Soup - Light "Angel Hair Nest" Soup

Σούπα Φιδές

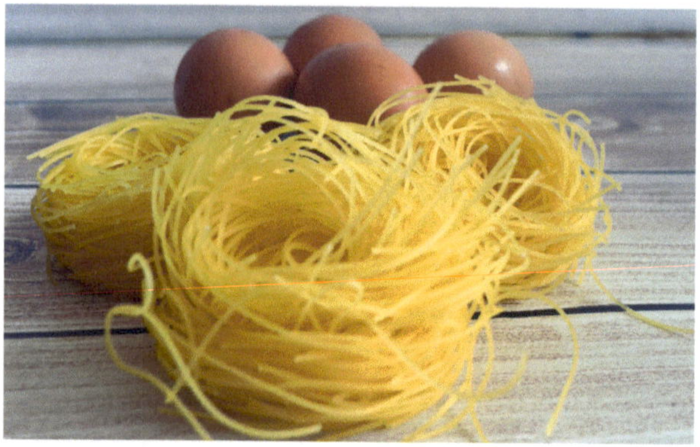

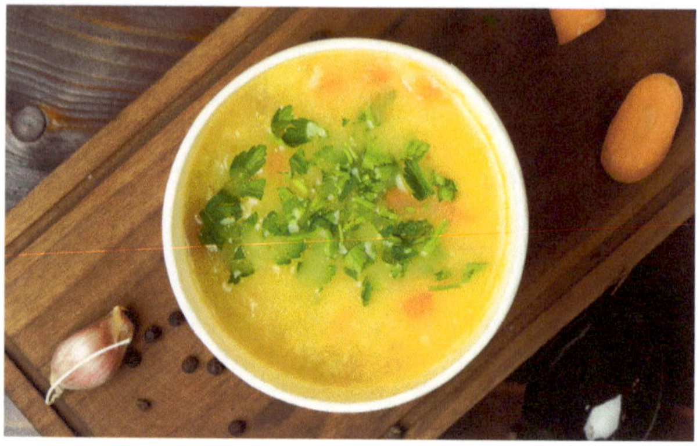

This soup is very light and we often make it when our health is compromised and we need a light broth and cannot digest much else. You can make a quick batch when you just want something warm in your tummy. You could call this the Greek simple version of ramen noodles. This soup is what my kids ask for when they are not feeling well, even to this day. The cracked pepper in this soup is a great immune booster, as is the fresh olive oil and freshly squeezed lemon juice.

- 2 Angel Hair Nests
- 6 cups water or chicken broth
- 4 green onions sliced
  - Salt + Pepper to taste
- 1 juice of lemon

In a large pot bring water or broth to a boil. (Use water or vegetable broth for vegetarian version).

Add angel hair nests and cook for about 3 minutes.

Once pasta is cooked, add the onions and spices. Freshly cracked pepper is preferred in this recipe.

Mix in lemon juice and serve. Add salt as needed.

If you are not using this as a quick remedy, then feel free to add other light ingredients per your liking such as tofu, carrots, spinach, parsley, or even easier digestible proteins such as shrimp or chicken. A little bit of organic tomato paste will add some depth to it as well.

Serves 6 people ***(Autumn, Winter)***

Pair with: Enjoy by itself

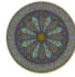

GF DF

Tas Kebab Soup or Stew - Hearty Beef Soup

I still remember one of the first times I prepared this meal and enjoyed it with a group of friends from high school. It is a meal of Persian origin, and is the combination of the beef stew and pilaf rice that makes this dish so popular. Its rich and deep taste is a meal that will leave you satisfied for a long time.

- ¼ cup olive oil
- 2.5 lbs. lean beef or lamb (either stew meat or cubed steak strips)
- 2 red bell peppers, coarsely chopped
- 1 yellow bell pepper, coarsely chopped
- 2 fresh tomatoes, chopped in squares
- 1 white/yellow onion, coarsely chopped
- 4 large carrots, sliced in thick rounds
- 4 celery ribs, chopped in large chunks
- 4 cups of organic beef bone broth
- 3 cups filtered water
- ½ cup loosely chopped fresh parsley
- 2 tsps. dried oregano
- ½ tsp. season salt
- • Pepper to taste

Combine cubed beef, red and yellow peppers, and chopped onion in a bowl. Dress with salt, pepper, season salt and oregano and toss to coat and mix well. Cover and let stand in the fridge for at least 1 hour.

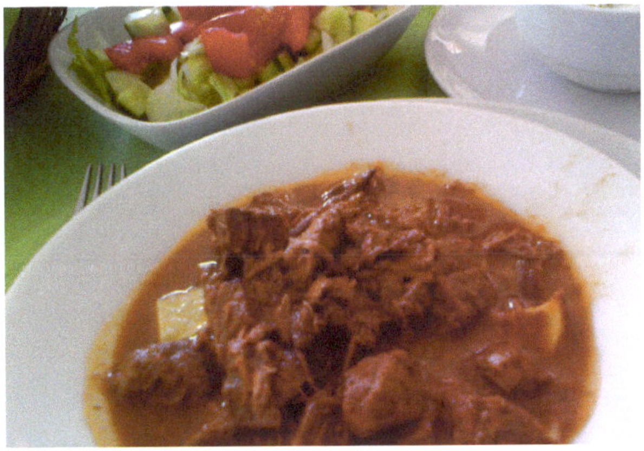

Add olive oil to large pot and sauté beef mixture until beef is well browned and vegetables are softened.

Add carrots and sauté for a couple of minutes, then add celery bits and do the same.

Add bone broth and water to pot and bring to a boil. Cook in med/low heat with a lid for 20 minutes.

Add chopped parsley and cook for another minute. Taste soup and add salt/pepper as needed.

This dish is typically served on top of rice pilaf and is mixed in with the sauce from the stew to create a unique combination.

Serves 6 people *(Autumn, Winter)*

Pair with: Rice Pilaf. Make a bed of white Rice pilaf and ladle the beef stew over the rice.

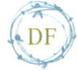

DF GF

Warm and Soothing - Soups

Watercress Chicken Soup

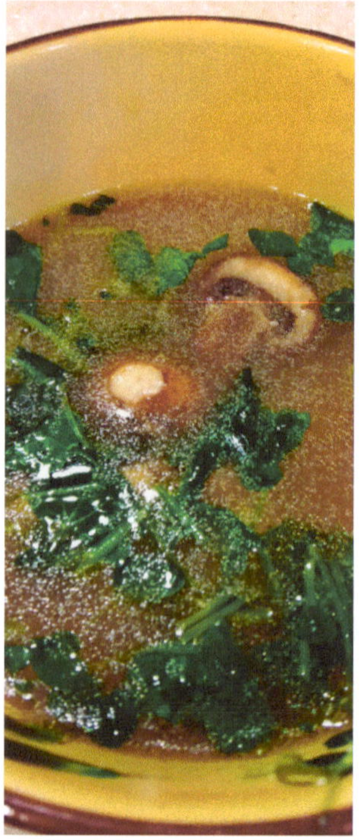

This simple and tasty recipe has been with me since my college days. It was something I could whip up really fast and had a bit of substance to it. While watercress is not always easy to find, when late winter/ early spring would come around, it would show up in the market again. That was my cue to once again prepare this delicately tasting soup. This was my ramen version for a quick but nutritious meal.

Watercress is a soft leafy green vegetable that often is found growing close to natural springs. It seems it was famed to have been one of the favorite wild medicinals used by Hippocrates, deemed "father of modern medicine." He was purportedly said to have built his first hospital by a natural spring-fed stream filled with fresh watercress to help heal and treat his patients. Even to this day it is often used as an herbal remedy for the treatment of scurvy, arthritis, gout and coughs.

As a nutrient-rich wild food source, it has been utilized for its nutritious leafy stems, as both a raw vegetable and steamed green. Its taste is a bit spicy, similar to arugula, but much smoother.

- ¼ cup olive oil
- 2.5 lbs. chicken breast, cubed
- 16 oz. mini portabella mushrooms, sliced
- ¼ cup sherry for taste
- 4 cups organic chicken stock
- 2 cups water
- 2 cups fresh watercress, loosely chopped
  - Salt + pepper to taste

In a large pot sauté chicken cubes in olive oil until lightly browned.

Add mushroom slices and sauté until they are softened. Pour in sherry and mix well to cover the chicken. Add chicken broth and water and bring to boil. Cook on medium fire for about 10 minutes.

Season to taste with salt and pepper

Add chopped watercress and cook for another minute and then remove the pot from the fire. Taste soup and add salt/pepper as needed.

Serves 6 people *(Autumn, Winter)*

Pair with: White Rice or just enjoy by itself

GF DF

Yuvarlakia - Traditional Greek Meatball Soup

Γιουβαρλάκια

Everybody in our family loves this soup! Easy to make and so tasty with its lemon egg sauce, it is sure to please all.

- 1.5 lbs. of minced beef
- 1 onion minced
- 2 garlic gloves, minced
- ½ cup parsley, finely chopped
- 1 tbsp. fresh mint, chopped
- 1 tsp. dry oregano
- 1 cup basmati rice
- 1 egg yolk
- 1 tsp. salt
- 4 tbsps. olive oil
- ½ cup gluten Free flour or Rice flour
- 2-3 eggs, in room temperature for "Avgolemono" sauce
- 1-2 large lemons, juiced
    - Add salt to taste

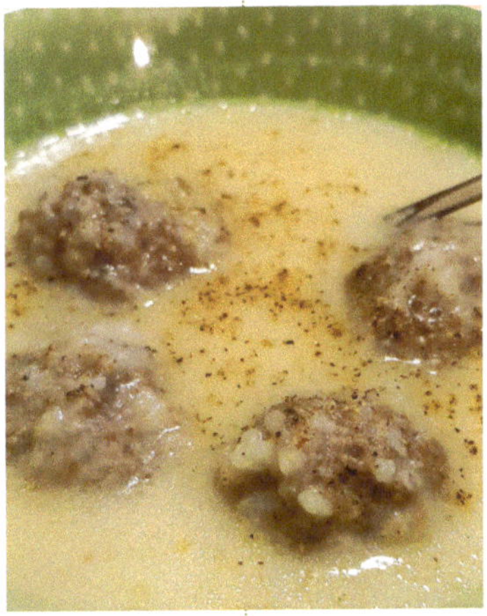

In a large bowl combine minced meat with onion, garlic, herbs, rice, egg and spices until well blended. Make small meatballs and roll in gluten free flour. In a large pot, bring water and olive oil to boil, enough to cover all meatballs as you add them to the pot. Bring to boil and immediately lower fire to a simmer for about 25 to 30 minutes, until meat is cooked and rice is tender. If necessary add more water during cooking time.

Meanwhile prepare "Avgolemono" sauce. Avgolemono sauce is one of the most traditional soup sauces in Greece. It is a mix of raw egg and lemon combined with the liquid that is being cooked. It is best prepared right before the dish is ready. Take the two eggs that have been in room temperature and beat together in a medium sized bowl, until they are pale and foamy. Continuing to beat eggs, slowly drizzle in fresh lemon juice until well mixed. Then slowly take 2 to 3 ladlefuls of the warm soup and begin drizzling into egg mixture, while still continuing to blend. You want to do this slowly in order to avoid the egg from turning as you add the hot liquid in. When the meatballs are ready, remove pot from fire and slowly pour in avgolemono sauce while gently stirring the pot. Sprinkle with extra fresh parsley if you like and serve while warm.

Serves 6 people *(Autumn, Winter)*

Pair with: This is served as a main dish and in Greece this is often enjoyed with some white crisp wine.

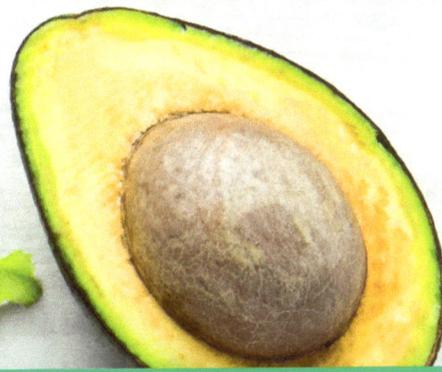

4

Crisp and Crunchy
Fresh Salads

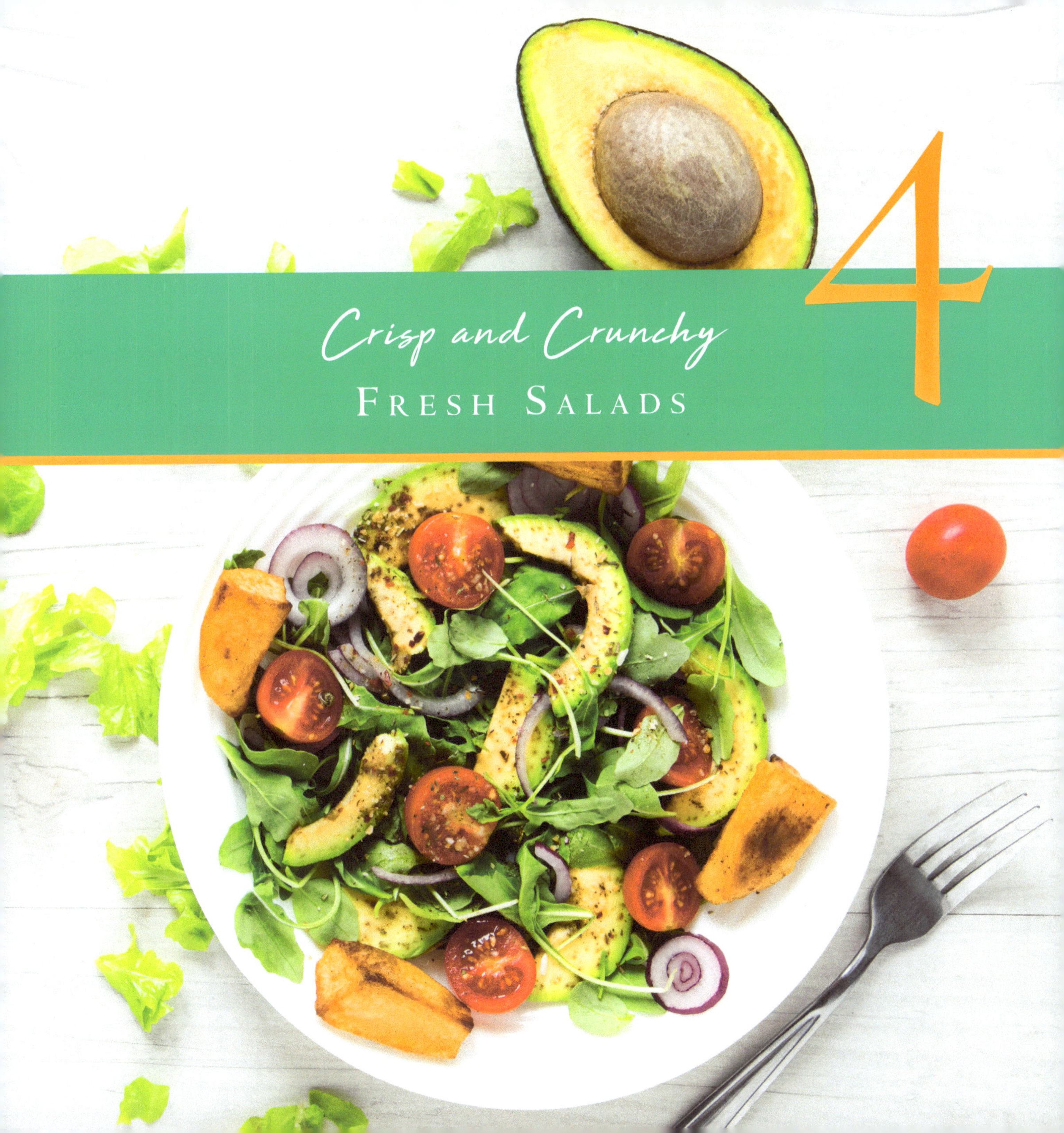

GF V

Arugula with Roquefort Salad - A spicy & deep flavored salad

Ρόκα με ροκφόρ

In our neck of the woods in Northern Colorado, arugula comes up first thing in the spring while the weather is still a little crisp. Take note that if you are growing your own arugula, the acidity of the soil will give a stronger or milder flavor to this green.

This is one of my favorite salads, as it signals the beginning of warmer weather and our garden coming back to bloom from the cold winter months.

- 3 cups of fresh arugula greens
- ¼ cup finely chopped green onions
- ¼ cup chopped walnuts
- 6 oz. crumbled Roquefort cheese
- ⅓ cups olive oil
- 3 tbsp. red wine vinegar
  - Salt + Pepper to taste

Place fresh arugula in a bowl and add finely chopped green onions and toss. Top with Roquefort cheese and walnuts.

Mix dressing in a separate small bowl, adding oil, vinegar, salt and pepper and then drizzle lightly over the salad.

Serves 4 people ***(Spring, Summer)***

Pair with: Any grilled meat dish or serve as a light lunch.

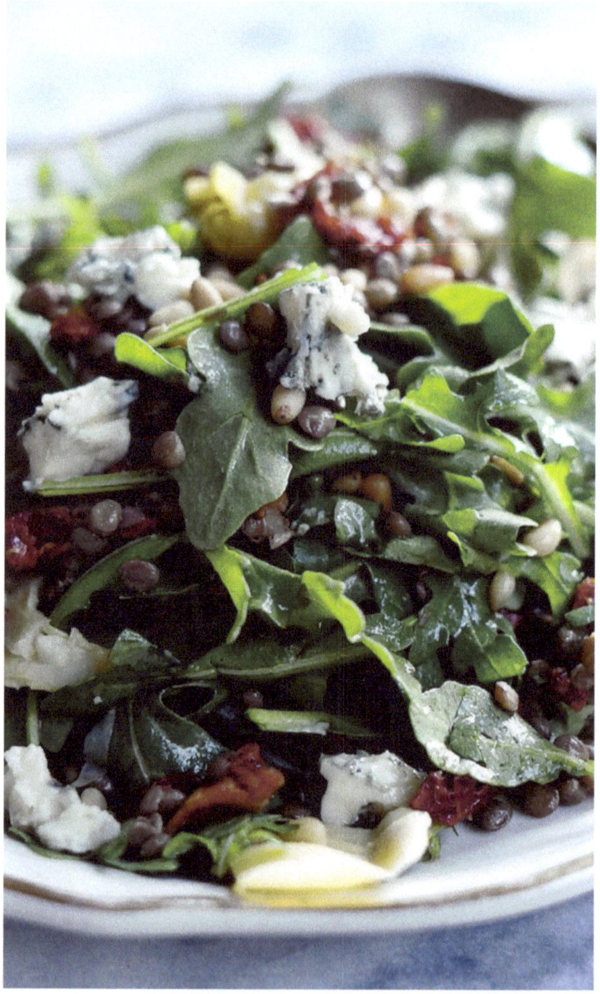

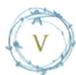

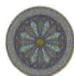

DF GF V

Cabbage Salad - Easy, Fresh & With A Tang

Λαχανοσαλάτα

Perfect as a side dish, our whole family enjoys the freshness of this salad. While cabbage takes a while to mature on the plant, the end results is a tightly woven crisp medley of leaves that will leave your mouth craving more. The addition of rice vinegar in this recipe accentuates this crispness and awakens your taste buds. This is a cold weather vegetable and it ushers the feeling of fresh veggies into the winter months.

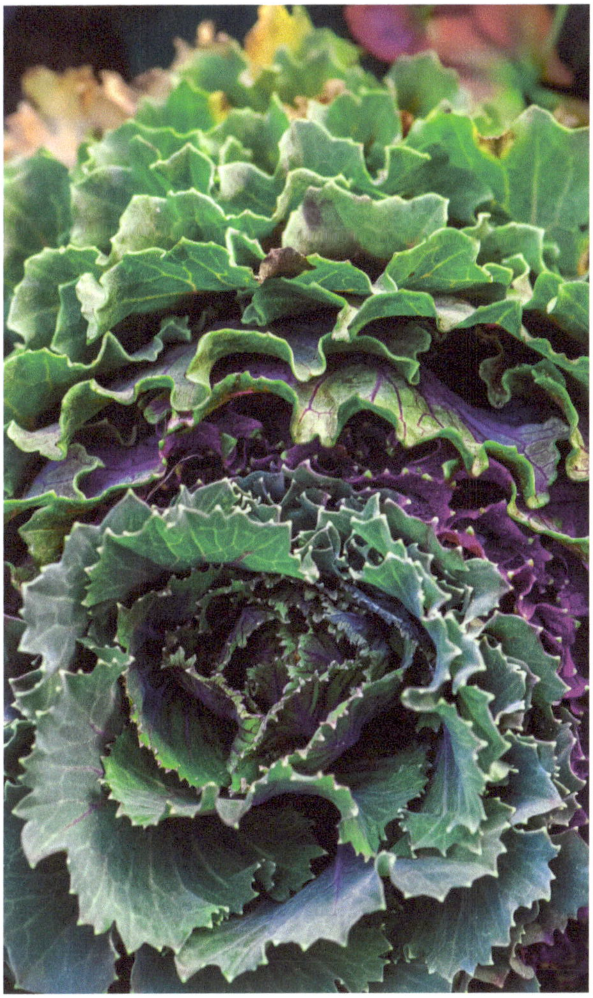

- ½ head of green cabbage
- ⅓ head of red cabbage
- 3 green onions, chopped fine
- 1 tbsp. olive oil
- 1 tbsp. white rice vinegar
- 1 tsp. black & white toasted sesame seeds
  - Salt + Pepper to taste

Slice the cabbage heads very fine and place in a medium bowl. Finely chop green onions and add to bowl.

Add olive oil, rice vinegar, salt and pepper and gently toss salad. Sprinkle sesame seeds on top.

Serves 4 people ***(Summer, Autumn, Winter)***

Pair with: Any grilled meat dish or as a light lunch

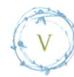

DF GF V

Caprese Salad

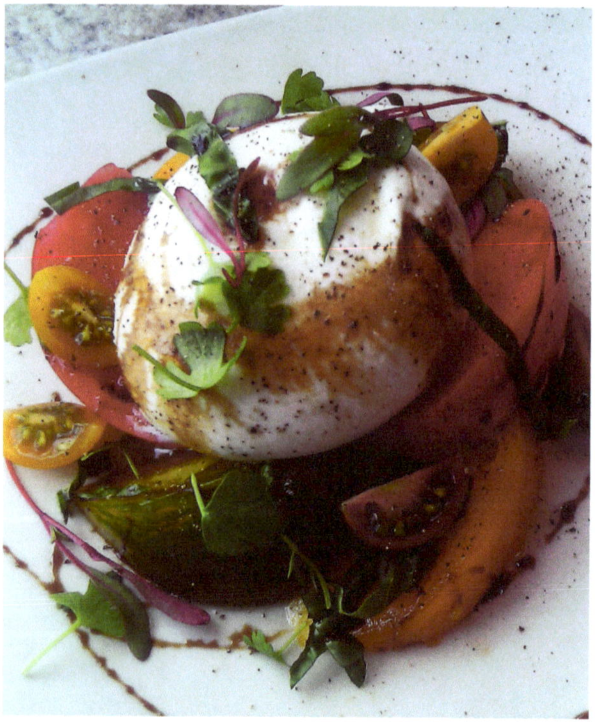

This is such a simple salad bursting with taste! Although dairy has long ago left my diet, this classic Italian salad has left a fond memory on my taste buds. Recently I discovered a vegan cheese that works rather well in this recipe, so if you follow a dairy fee diet, all is not lost. Search your local market for plant alternatives to cheese.

This salad is easy and fast to prepare with colorful red, white and green tones. Heirloom tomatoes are wonderful in this combination if you have access to them. The mozzarella cheese can either be cut in slices and snuck in between the tomatoes or placed in the middle of the serving plate. Large basil leaves add their aroma in this mix. The capers add a delicious touch to this dish and a lingering aftertaste that makes one wish for more. Capers grow wild in Greece between the stone steps and in dry patches of land. We harvest them in the summer and pickle them for use throughout the year.

- 5 large tomatoes, sliced thin
- 6 oz. sliced mozzarella or dairy free alternative
- 20 whole basil leaves, washed
- 2 tbsp. capers
- 2 tbsp. olive oil
- 1 tbsp. balsamic vinegar
- • Salt + Pepper to taste

The classic way to arrange a Caprese salad is to layer the mozzarella, tomato and basil in a ring or row. Ideally, the finished dish will showcase a beautiful palette of red, green and white, whether you lay it out on a platter or in a bowl. Drizzle olive oil, vinegar and salt and pepper. Serve immediately.

Serves 6 people *(Summer, Autumn)*

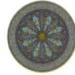

DF GF V

Carrot Salad

Σαλάτα καρότο

Such a simple but delightful salad, nutritious and light. Easy and fast to prepare with colorful orange and green tones. When I was growing up, there was a restaurant around the corner from where we lived that used to serve a carrot salad with a special white dressing that had me mesmerized. That was the beginning of my love affair with carrot salad!

- 5 large carrots, grated
- ¼ cup chopped carrot greens
- 4 green onions, finely diced
- 2 bunches of fresh dill, finely chopped

Dressing

- 1″ fresh ginger root, grated
- ½ lemon, squeezed
- ¼ cup olive oil
- 4 tbsps. rice vinegar
    - Salt + Pepper to taste

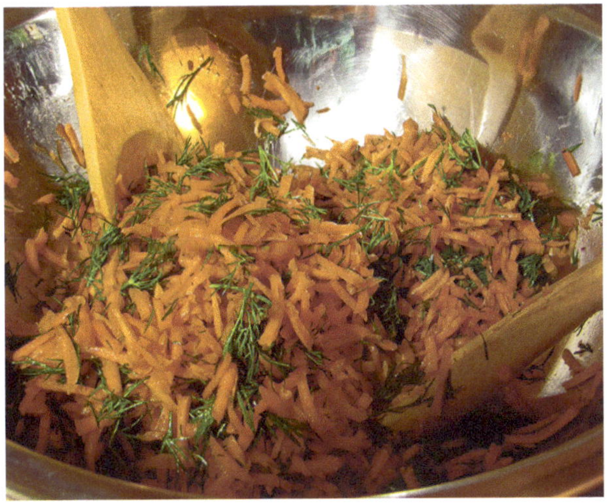

In a bowl add all the ingredients and toss before dressing salad.

Blend all dressing ingredients and mix well together. Pour over salad and blend. Serve immediately.

Serves 6 people ***(Summer, Autumn, Winter)***

Pair with: as a salad side dish or with any kind of protein. Goes well with beef, chicken and fish of your choice.

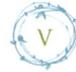

DF GF V

Cauliflower & Green Olive Salad

This creation came about from using what was available in the fridge one day and quickly has become a favorite. It is loaded with nutritional value and great taste and can easily be served as a main dish for lunch or dinner, as it is so filling.

- ½ large cauliflower, chopped in small bites
- 1 cup mixed greens
- ½ cup roasted red peppers, sliced
- ½ cup sun dried tomatoes, sliced
- ½ small red onion, sliced fine
- 10 green pimiento olives, sliced
- ½ cup Kalamata olives, sliced
- 2 tbsp. olive oil
- 1 tbsp. red wine vinegar
  - Salt + Pepper to taste
  - Dash of oregano
  - Sprig of parsley for garnish or in salad

Mix all ingredients and toss gently.

Add olive oil, red wine vinegar, salt and pepper and oregano and gently toss salad before serving. The secret here is in the red vinegar. Make sure you use a good quality, aged, red wine vinegar which brings out the taste in the veggies.

Serves 4 people ***(Summer, Autumn)***

Pair with: as a side dish or by itself.

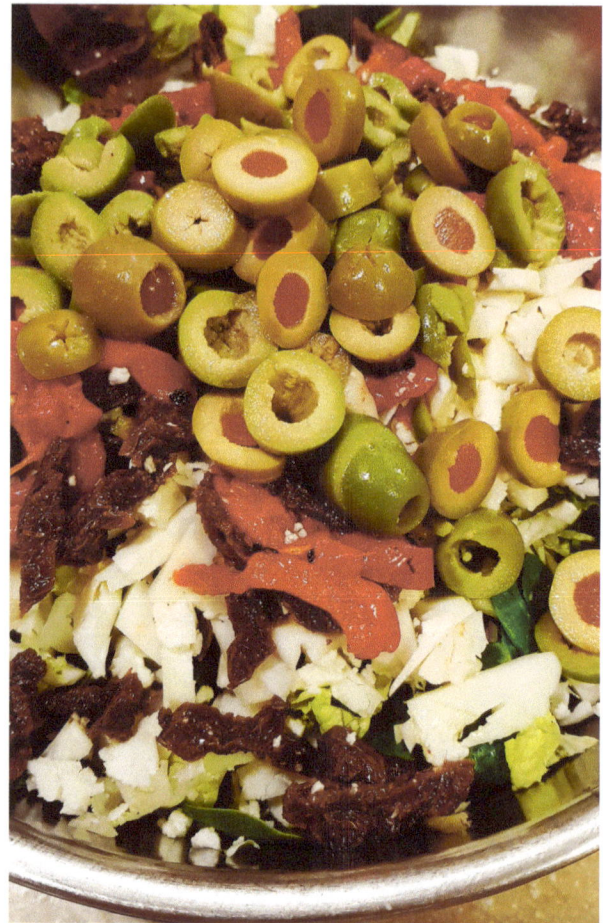

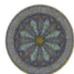

DF GF V

Corinna's Pico de Gallo Explosion

This combination is one of my favorites, not only to eat as a salad but also to use as a garnish for meat dishes, such as skirt steak or as an appetizer scooped with chips. When paired with any protein main dish, it brings a certain freshness to the palette and aids in digestion. Pico is best made with ripe but firm tomatoes; roma tomatoes can be great here as they are easy to dice without being mushed.

At times I will also use color heirloom tomatoes from our garden before they get too soft. I do prefer English cucumber in most of my salads, as they do not have as many seeds and have a great crisp taste to them. Armenian cucumbers are another option in this salad, although may be a bit bitter in taste.

- 5 large ripe but firm tomatoes, diced
- 1 large diced English cucumber
- 2 firm but not hard avocados, diced
- ½ red onion, finely diced
- 1 small jalapeno, diced
- ⅓ cup finely chopped cilantro

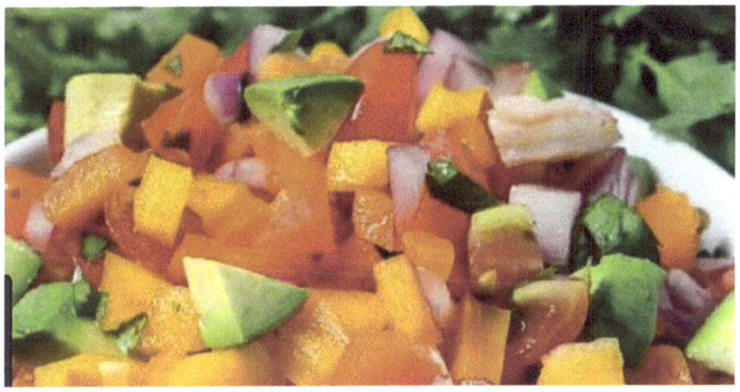

Dressing

- ⅓ cup rice wine vinegar
- ½ cup olive oil
- 1/8 tsp. pequin pepper flakes (optional)
  - Salt + Pepper to taste

In a bowl add all the ingredients and toss before dressing salad. Blend all dressing ingredients and mix well together. Pour over salad and blend.

Serves 6 people ***(Summer, Autumn)***

Pair with: as a side dish or garnish for meat dishes or by itself, perhaps even with some organic corn chips.

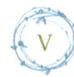

DF GF V

Crisp and Crunchy - Fresh Salads

Crisp Cucumber Salad - Easy, Fresh & Crisp Salad. Perfect For A Side Dish

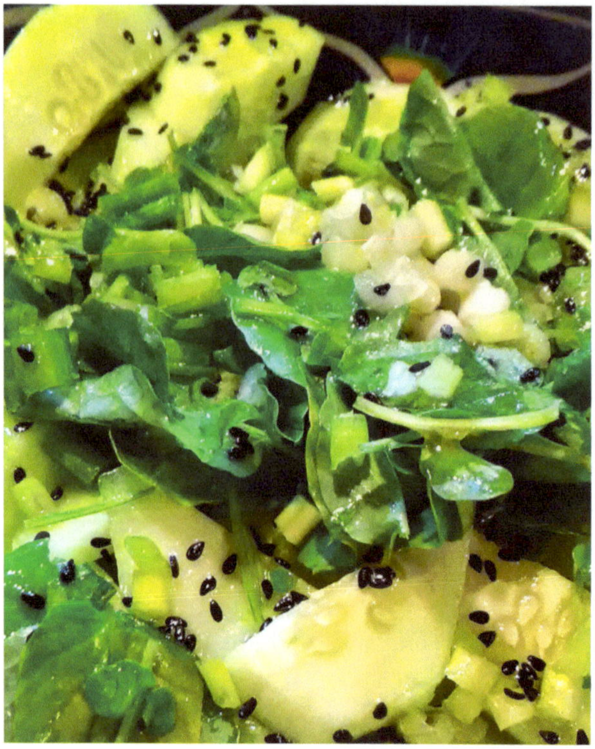

Sometimes we have such an abundance of cucumbers in the garden, and a simple crisp salad is all we need for lunch. The English type cucumbers are crunchy and have few seeds. They do really well with the soy sauce as they do not become soggy. Try them and you will not be sorry. This is such a wonderful salad for a light meal.

- 2 large English cucumbers
- 1 cup watercress
- 1 tbsp. olive oil
- 1 tbsp. Tamari free soy sauce
- 1 tbsp. black sesame seeds

Cut cucumbers in long diagonal thick slices. Cut stems off watercress and mix with cucumbers in a bowl. Mix olive oil and soy sauce and pour over cucumbers. Mix together. Sprinkle black sesame seeds on top and serve.

Serves 4 people ***(Summer, Autumn)***

Pair with: Light pasta dish, Asian flavored dishes.

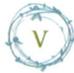

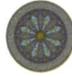

DF GF V

Cruciferous Salad with Turmeric Dressing

An incredible mix of crunchy veggies that brings freshness to your mouth. Unique spices create the delicious and healthful dressing that brings a kick to this recipe.

Pairs beautifully with steak, or other protein to your liking.

- ½ green cabbage, thinly sliced
- ½ red cabbage, thinly sliced
- 1 bunch of Russian kale, torn in small pieces
- 1 cup thinly sliced or shredded Brussel sprouts
- ½ tsp. organic turmeric powder
- ½ tsp. organic ginger powder
- 2 tbsp. olive oil
- 1 tbsp. apple cider vinegar
  - Sea salt + cracked pepper to taste

In a small container mix olive oil, apple cider vinegar and spices until they are well blended. Mix all veggies together in a large bowl, top with dressing and gently toss salad before serving.

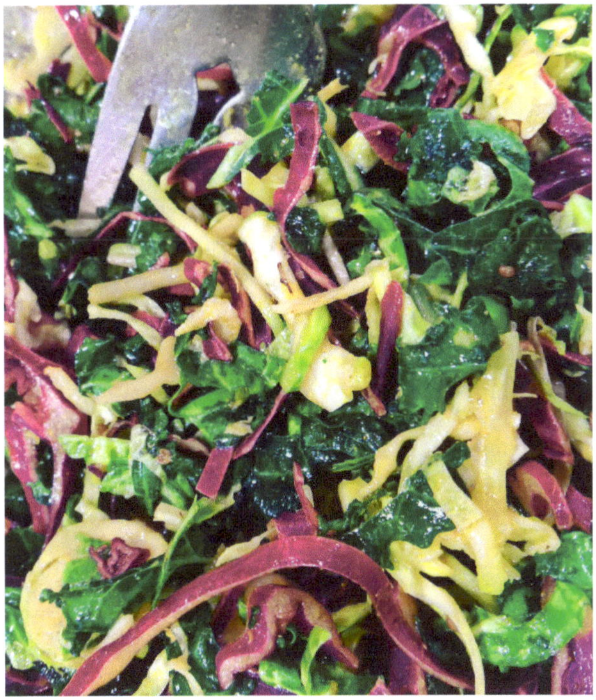

Serves 4 people ***(Autumn, Winter)***

Pair with: as a side dish or by itself.

DF GF V

Cucumber Sumac Salad

This is such a simple crunchy salad and adds a touch of freshness to any meal. Salads are my favorite go to, and I often feel that a meal is not complete without some fresh veggies. I prefer English or Armenian cucumbers that have less seeds in them and a unique crunch as you bite into them. Peel the skin of the cucumber lengthwise every other row and you create a nice design as you cut them into rounds.

The peppers that I used on this salad are also very unique, not only in their taste, but also their look. They are a variegated type of yellow/red bell peppers with a smooth taste. Sumac is a tart and dark red spice commonly found in the Mediterranean cuisine that lends a very unique taste. You can usually find it online or in Mediterranean markets.

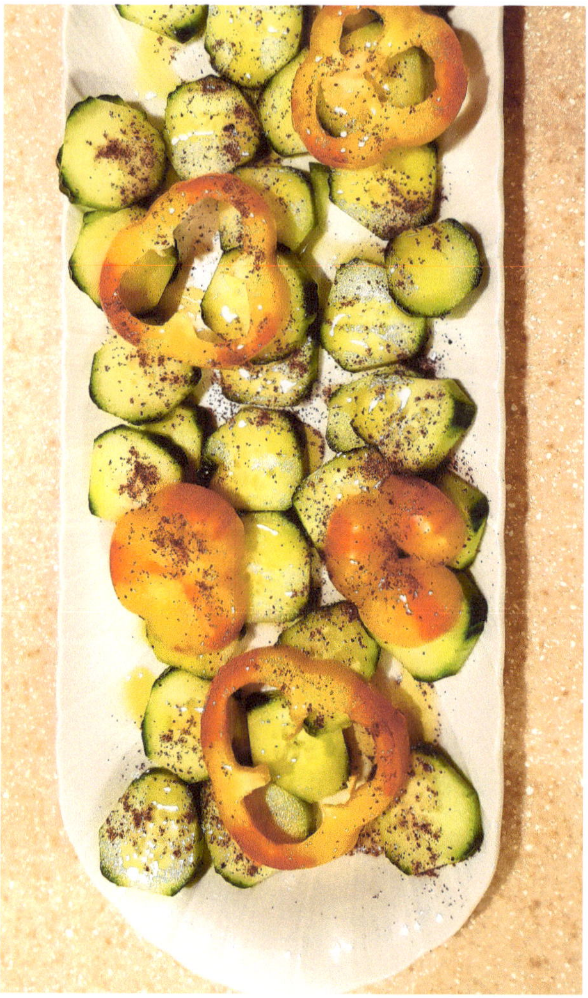

- 1 large English type cucumber cut in round slices
- ½ yellow/red variegated bell pepper cut in slices
- 2 tbsp. olive oil
- 1 tsp. red wine vinegar
- 1 tsp. sumac seasoning
- Sea salt + cracked pepper to taste

Cut cucumbers and peppers either in a bowl or flat dish. Sprinkle with olive oil, red vinegar and spices and serve.

Serves 4 people ***(Summer, Autumn, Winter)***

GF V

Green Bean & Watermelon Salad

This salad is so wonderfully refreshing and light for the summer months! I remember from a young age combining watermelon and feta cheese, and it still is one of my favorite flavors. I usually wait for the middle of the season, as the watermelons become sweeter. Keep the watermelon in the fridge until you are ready to mix the salad for an explosion of taste and coolness!

Add the beans, and this truly is a meal in itself. The sweetness of the watermelon pairs so well with the astringent nature of the beans that it makes this combination a winner. Since many of our family members have dairy allergies, we serve the feta cheese on the side but you can crumble it on top and lightly mix before serving.

- 1 lb. of French string beans, steamed
- 2 cups, chopped watermelon
- ½ cup of halved walnuts
- ¾ cup crumbled, sheep's feta
- 2 tbsps. loosely chopped parsley

Top with Balsamic vinaigrette (see sauces).

Begin by washing the green beans under cold water, and then blanching them. You can steam them for about 5 minutes, then quickly immerse them in a bowl of ice water to stop the cooking process to maintain their natural deep green color. Add the beans to a large salad bowl and move on to the watermelon.

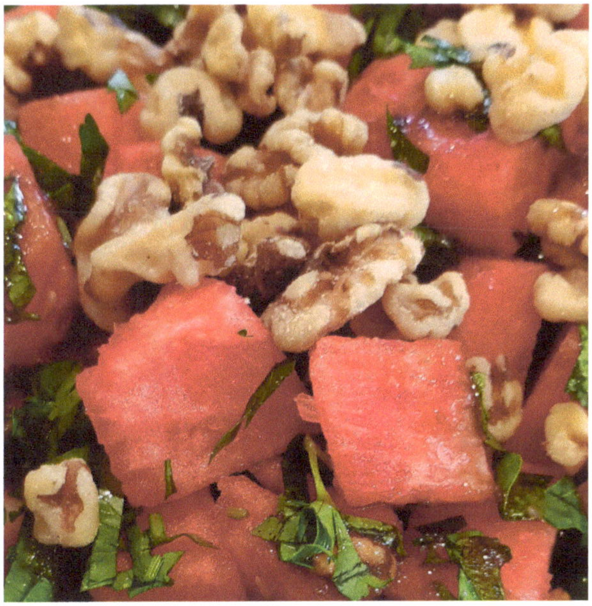

After you have cooled the fruit in the fridge, cut the watermelon in small, bitesize cubes and add them to the serving bowl.

Sprinkle with walnuts and crumbled feta cheese and then add loosely chopped parsley on top.

Pour on the dressing and you are ready to serve!

Serves 6 people ***(Spring, Summer)***

Pair with: Serve as a main dish for a light lunch.

GF V

Crisp and Crunchy - Fresh Salads

FETA & CHICKPEA SALAD

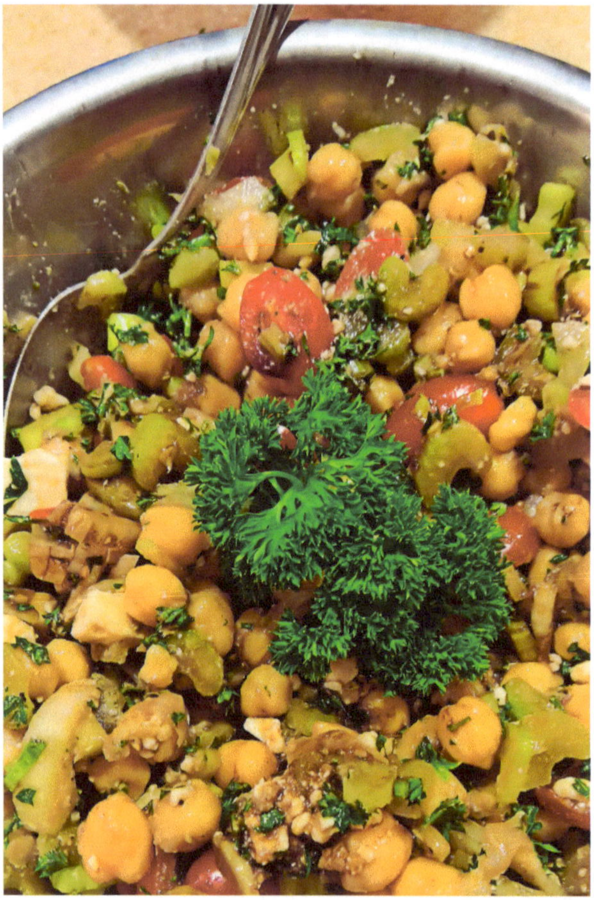

If you love feta cheese, this blend is incredible! Crunchy and soft at the same time, it is a bouquet of flavors that explode in your mouth.

- 2 15 oz. cans of chickpeas, drained of juices
- 8 large stalks of celery, chopped fine
- 1 ½ cup of halved cherry tomatoes
- ¾ cup crumbled, sheep's feta
- 6 tbsp. olive oil
- 4 tbsp. balsamic vinegar
- ⅓ cup, fresh chopped parsley (or 1 tbsp. dry parsley)
- ⅓ cup, fresh chopped thyme (or 1/2 tbsp. dry thyme)
  - Sea salt + cracked pepper to taste (feta is pretty salty, so use salt sparingly or not at all).

In a large container add the drained chickpeas, chopped celery, halved tomatoes and feta and mix well. Add olive oil, balsamic vinegar, salt and pepper and herbs and mix until they are well blended.

Serves 6 people ***(Autumn, Winter)***

Pair with: as a side dish or by itself.

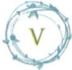

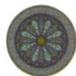

GF DF

"Horiatiki" Salad - Classic

Χωριάτικη Σαλάτα

Fresh and wholesome ingredients create this delicious salad which in Greece we refer to as the village salad or "Horiatiki". Perfect for a side dish or enjoy it as the main dish on a beautiful warm summer day. Feel free to omit the feta cheese or olives if not to your liking.

- 2 large sliced organic tomatoes
- 1 long English type cucumber
- 1 small red onion, sliced fine
- 1 thick slice of feta cheese
- ½ cup Kalamata olives
- 2 tbsp. olive oil
- 1 tbsp. red wine vinegar
  - Salt + Pepper to taste
  - Dash of oregano
  - Sprig of parsley for garnish or in salad

Gently slice your tomatoes and cucumber into a medium bowl. Finely slice the red onion and add to bowl. Toss in olives and top with whole slice of feta cheese or cube it and mix it into the salad.

Add olive oil, red wine vinegar, salt and pepper and oregano and gently toss salad before serving. Once again, the secret here is in the red vinegar. Make sure you use a good quality, aged, red wine vinegar which brings out the taste in the veggies.

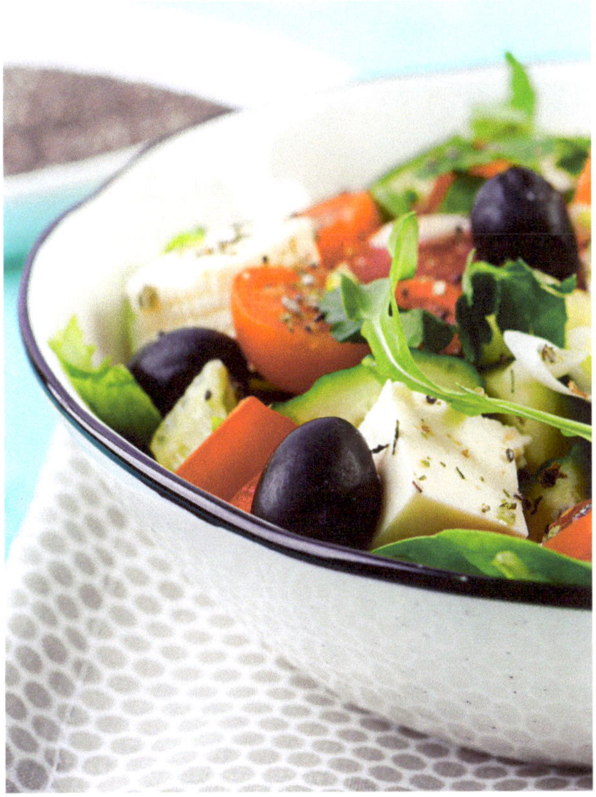

In some areas of Greece they add thinly sliced green peppers or romaine lettuce.

Serves 4 people ***(Summer, Autumn)***

Pair with: as a side dish or by itself.

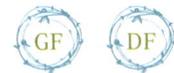

DF GF V

Crisp and Crunchy - Fresh Salads

Kale, Pear & Blueberry Salad

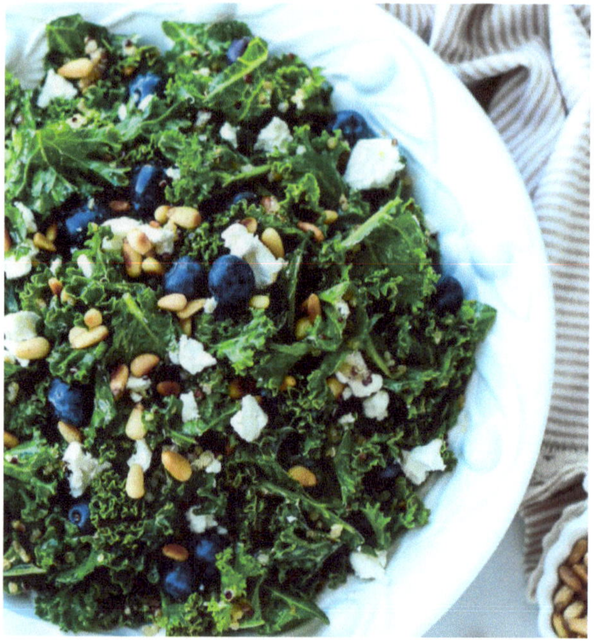

This is another one of those inspirations that came up in a moment's notice and literally from what was available in the fridge. Everybody in the family loves kale and this technique of preparing it for a salad gives it a whole other texture and taste. Kale is in the brassica family and is a great antioxidant, full of calcium, and vitamin C and K. The addition of some fruit in the salad kept it light and gave it a bit of sweetness. This fruit is more available later in the summer season for us as the blueberries and the pears will have a lot more flavor than produce grown in a greenhouse.

- 1 bunch, raw "Blue Night" Kale
- 8 leaves, Romaine lettuce, chopped fine
- ⅓ Beet, shredded
- 2 Green onions, thinly sliced
- 1 Asian pear, sliced thin
- ½ cup blueberries
- 1 tbsp. pine nuts
- ½ cup feta cheese - optional
- 4 tbsps. organic Olive Oil
- 2 tbsps. apple cider vinegar
- • Salt + Pepper to taste
- • Parsley, finely chopped for garnish

The trick here is to massage the fresh washed kale before mixing the salad. Add 1 tbsp. of olive oil to the raw kale in your bowl, and gently massage it with your hand until it becomes soft to the touch. This breaks down the veins which releases the flavor and makes it very palatable. Mix all remaining ingredients in order and dress with olive oil and vinegar.

Enjoy!

Serves 4 people *(Summer, Autumn, Winter)*

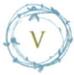

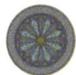

DF GF V

SPINACH - LEGUME SALAD

A healthy, effortless and nutritious salad.

Perfect for lunch or dinner.

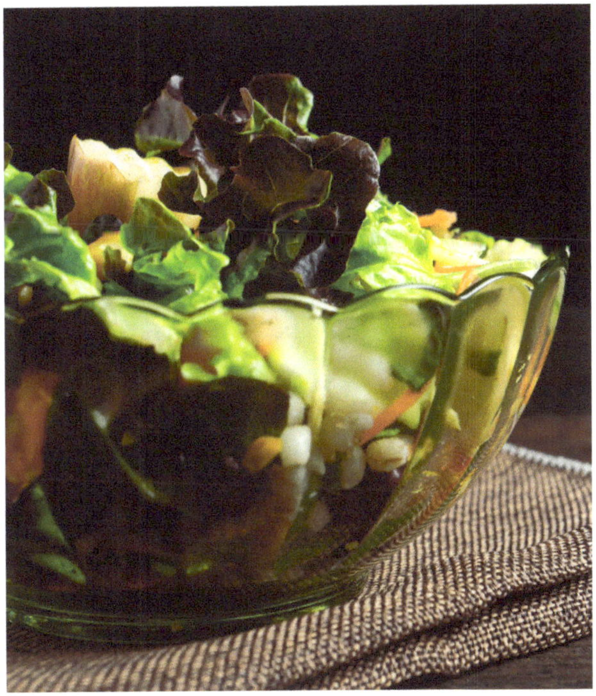

- 2 cups raw spinach or raw kale
- 1 cubed firm avocado
- ½ cup organic edamame beans
- 1 handful of sunflower seeds
- ¼ cup raisins or cran-raspberries
- 2 tbsp. organic olive oil
- 1 tbsp. lemon juice
- • Salt + Pepper to taste

Mix all ingredients in order and dress with olive oil or your favorite healthy salad dressing. Feel free to substitute beans with your favorite kind. Best with navy, garbanzo and white salad beans. You can also add or substitute finely chopped red cabbage, grapes or walnuts.

Serves 4 people ***(Spring, Summer)***

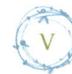

Spring Green Salad

This is a light mix of greens that is fresh, soft and crisp and is delightful for a day that you feel like something light in your tummy.

- ½ head finely chopped romaine lettuce
- 2.5 oz. baby lettuce leave mix, green/red
- ½ cup spinach leaves
- 1 English cucumber, quartered and sliced
- ½ cup of finely sliced colored bell peppers
- ⅓ cup finely sliced celery
- ⅓ cup finely sliced carrots
- 1 cup fresh snap peas
- 4 finely sliced green onions
- ⅓ cup, fresh chopped parsley
- 1 small tomato for garnish

Dressing

- ⅓ cup apple cider vinegar
- 2 tbsps. seed mustard of your liking
- ½ cup olive oil
  - Salt + Pepper to taste

In a bowl add all the ingredients and toss before dressing salad.

For dressing, first pour vinegar in small container, then add seed mustard and mix until well dissolved.

Add olive oil, salt and pepper, mix well and serve.

This salad is made with a mix of veggies that are grown through different seasons. Lettuce and spring greens, spinach and green onions usually start becoming available in the spring. Carrots, celery, cucumbers and peppers are usually available in late summer. Of course, with harvests being flown in from all around the world it is possible to have those available for most of the year. Their nutritional value however might not be the same according to how and where they were grown. Something to consider when you create such combinations.

Serves 6 people ***(Spring, Summer, Autumn, Winter)***

Pair with: as a side dish or by itself.

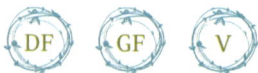

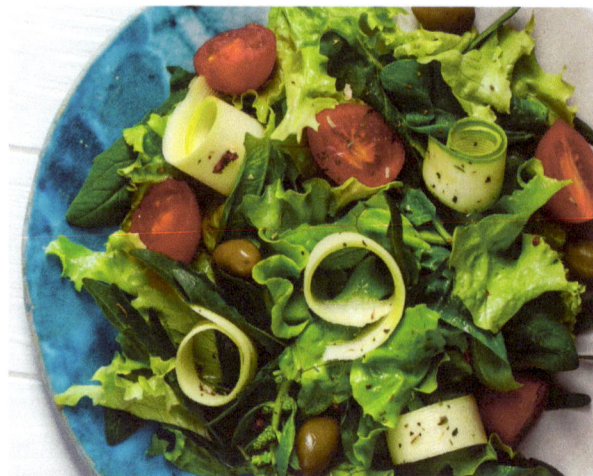

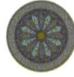

DF GF V

Tomato & Green Onion Salad

Easy, fresh and wholesome salad.
Perfect for a side dish.

5 large sliced organic tomatoes
cherry or heirloom tomatoes would be great too
3 green onions, chopped fine
1 tbsp. olive oil
1 tbsp. red wine vinegar
- Salt + Pepper to taste

Gently slice your tomatoes into a medium bowl. Finely chop green onions and add to bowl.

Add olive oil, red wine vinegar, salt and pepper and gently toss salad.

Serves 4 people ***(Summer, Autumn)***

Pair with: Oven roasted chicken or any grilled meat dish.

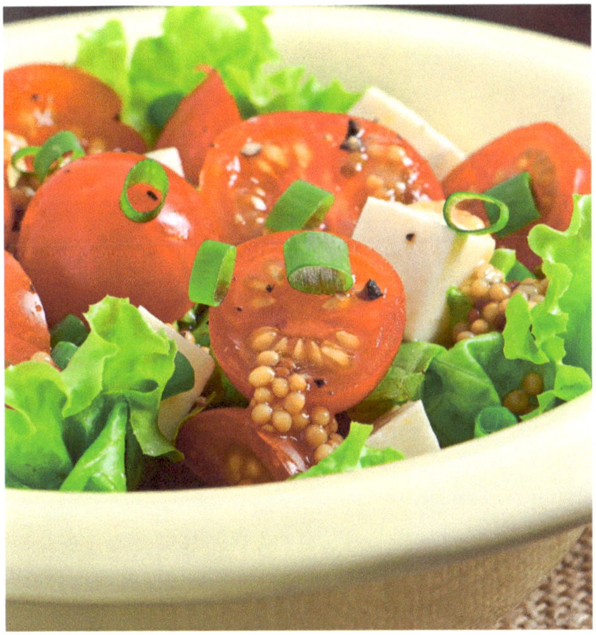

DF GF V

Potato Salad

Πατατοσαλάτα

Potato Salad – a Greek version of this filling recipe that makes a great side dish as well.

2 lbs. small red potatoes, boiled and halved
8 green onions, washed and sliced or
1 medium red onion, thinly chopped and diced
½ cup fresh parsley, finely chopped
½ cup Vegenaise (or mayonnaise) (optional)
4 tbsps. olive oil
2 tbsps. red wine vinegar

- Salt + Pepper to taste
- Kalamata olives or parsley for garnish

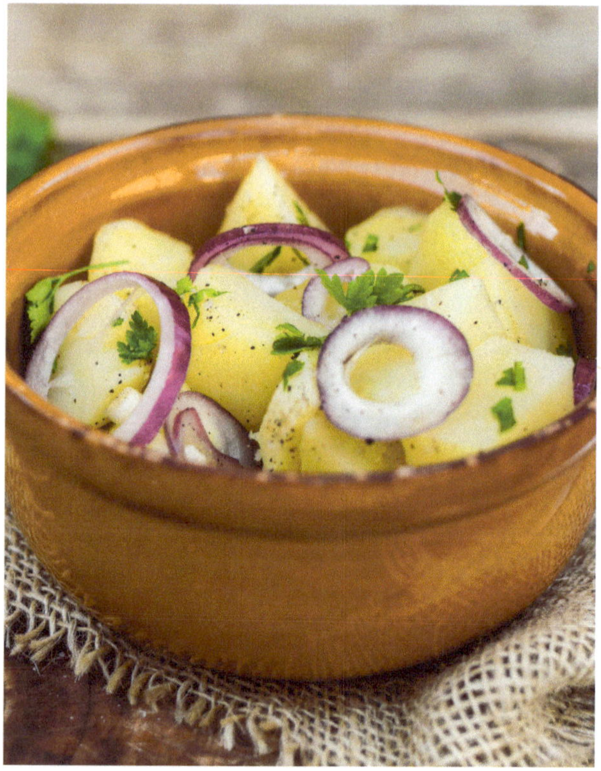

Combine firmly boiled and cut potatoes and green onions in a medium bowl. Prepare dressing in a separate small bowl and then pour over potatoes. Mix well and top with Kalamata olives or a sprig of fresh parsley.

Serves 6 people ***(Summer, Autumn, Winter)***

Pair with: grilled meat & fish dishes, barbeque.

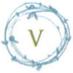

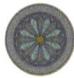

DF GF V

Beet salad

Παντζαροσαλάτα

A nutritious and delicious approach to beets, using leaves and bulbs.

6 large beets – 1 bunch with leaves, any color

Dressing

⅓ cup red wine vinegar

½ cup olive oil

1 large garlic glove, minced (optional)

3 tbsps. capers (optional)

- Salt + Pepper to taste

Prepare beets by cutting off bulbs, washing, scrubbing and peeling any rough skin off. Wash greens and set aside. If beets are really large, cut in half or quarter before adding to pot. Beets can take a long time to cook so I prefer to prepare mine in the pressure cooker which takes about 8 minutes.

Otherwise, place beet bulbs in a medium pot covered with water, bring to boil and cook 20 to 30 minutes until almost done. Add leaves and cook with the bulbs for another 5 minutes.

While still warm, place beets and leaves in a serving bowl. Meanwhile, preparing dressing by mixing all ingredients and then pour over warm beets.

Serves 6 people ***(Summer, Autumn, Winter)***

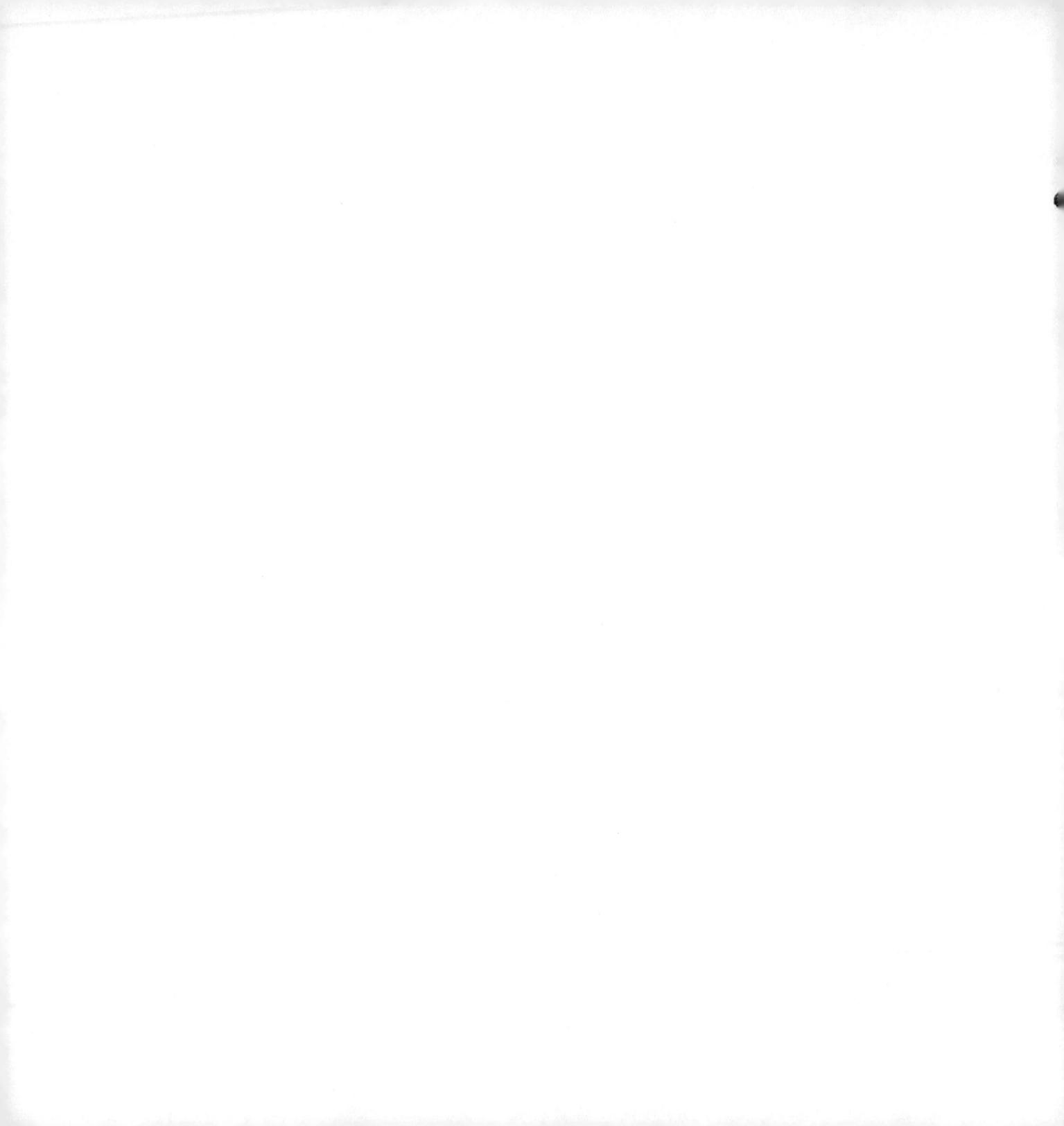

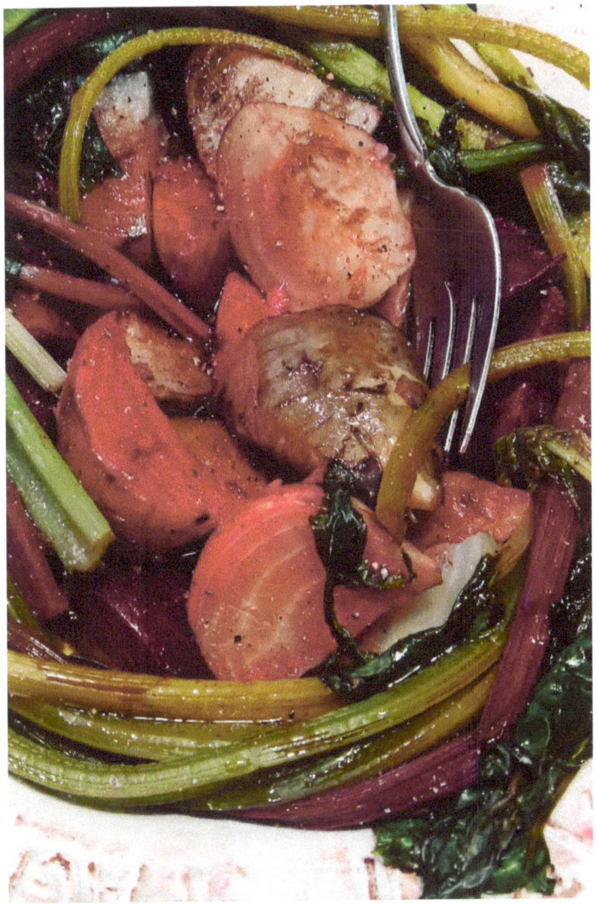

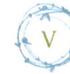

Pair with: as a warm side dish or a salad.

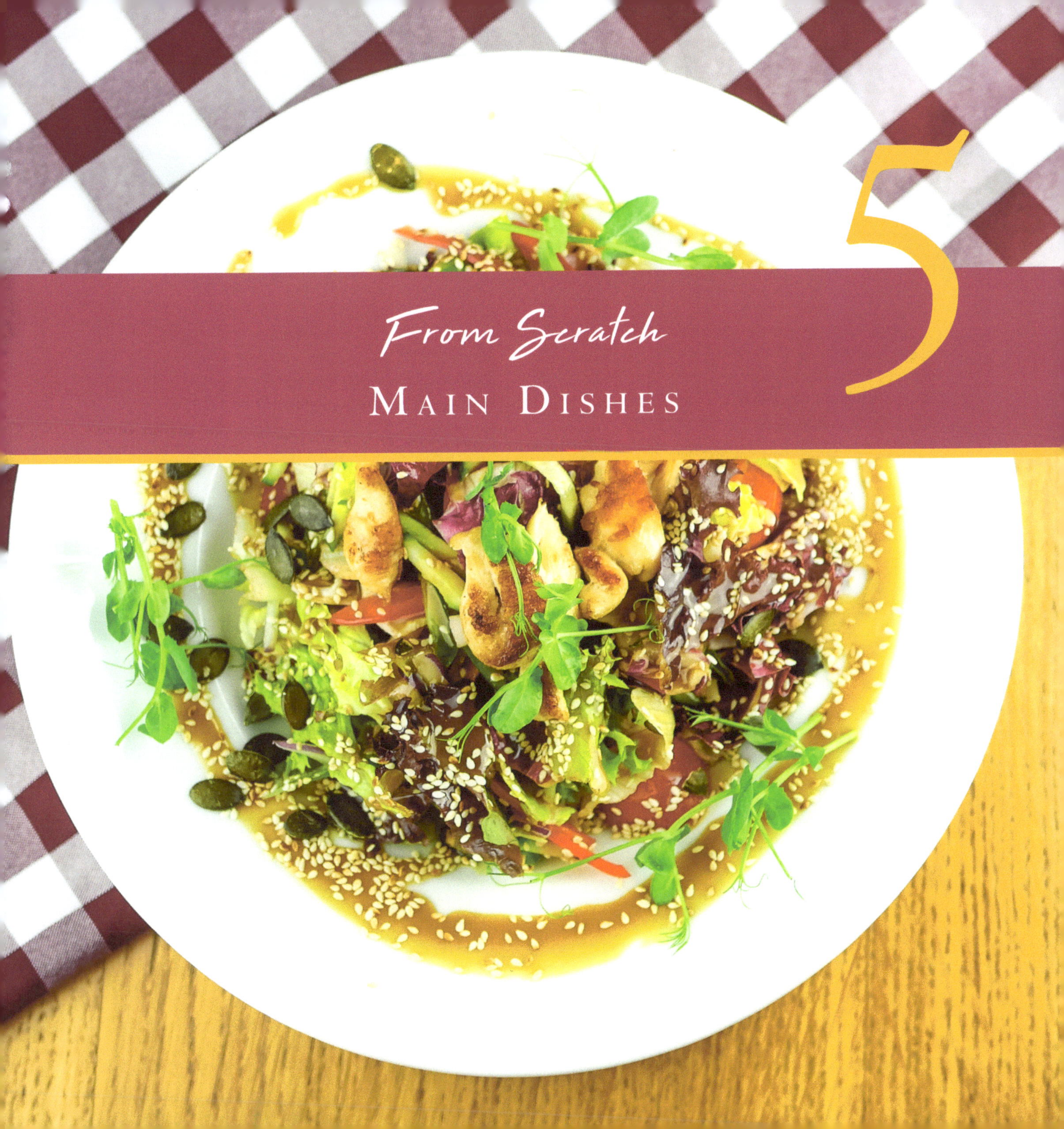

5 Main Dishes

DF GF

BEEF HAMBURGERS

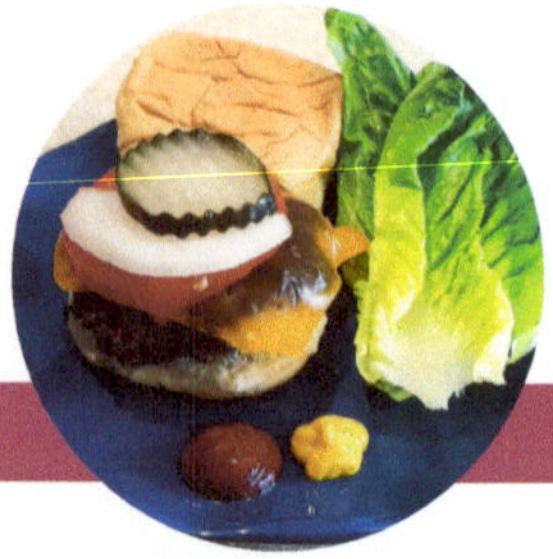

Hamburgers, as you can imagine are not a Mediterranean dish; we often make a similar version called Keftedes. However, here in the states hamburgers are a common meal and in our family we do indulge in this meal once in a while. As such my burger recipes are usually very involved but I was in a hurry one day and came up with this fast but still delicious and healthy recipe that stole our hearts.

- 4 lbs. organic beef (96% lean)
- 1 tbsp. season salt (I prefer Simply Organic brand)
- 1 tbsp. coconut aminos (in the soy section)
- 1 tbsp. dried organic parsley
- 6 slices of sharp cheddar cheese

For the garnish:

- 6 artisan baked hamburger buns, sliced in half cross length
- 6 romaine lettuce leaves
- 1 organic tomato, sliced
- 1 small red onion sliced
  - Ketchup and mustard to your liking

For the side dish:

- 2 ripe organic tomatoes, sliced in 4 wedges
- 1 12 oz. can of hearts of palm
- 1 tbsp. Greek olive oil
  - Sea salt to taste

In a large stainless steel bowl mix beef, season salt, coconut aminos and parsley until they are all well blended. Make six equal sized large patties out of the mixture. First make a ball out of your meat mixture and then add it to a stainless steel pan and flatten to ¼ inch thickness before cooking.

Place pan in the oven and cook burgers under low broil for about 15 minutes, turning the burgers once after 7 minutes. Burgers should be nicely browned on top. At the end of the 15 minutes, turn the oven off, pull oven grill out, place a slice of cheese on each burger, return grill to oven and let stand for about 3 minutes to melt. At the same time add bread buns in the oven to warm up. Then remove pan and buns out of the oven, place on stove top and serve burgers on buns.

Layer your hamburger buns with lettuce, tomato, onion, and condiments and set on large serving plate. Add 2 quartered tomatoes on the side of each burger, slice the heart of palm lengthwise and place next to tomatoes. Sprinkle with olive oil and salt and serve.

Serves 6 people *(All Seasons)*

Pair with: A simple green salad such as lettuce and green onions would pair nicely.

* For a gluten free version, use gluten free hamburger buns instead.

** For a dairy free version, replace cheese with vegan slices of cheese or omit altogether.

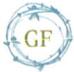

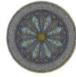

GF DF

Breaded Sole Fish

Ψάρι «Γλώσσα»

Delicate filets of fish.

2	lbs. fresh sole fish filets
4	eggs, lightly beaten
2	cups regular or gluten free bread crumbs
	Salt + Pepper to taste
1	cup Safflower oil or other high heat oil

Tartar Dressing

¾	cup Vegenaise
2	tbsp. olive oil
1	tsp lemon juice
1	tbsp. pickle relish
	Salt + Pepper

Side

16	oz. fresh baby spinach or salad mix
1/3	cup shredded parmesan cheese
2	tsps. Olive oil
	Drizzle fresh squeezed lemon juice
	Salt + Pepper to taste

Prepare two shallow dishes, one with beaten eggs and one with bread crumbs. Add salt and pepper into dish with breading and mix. Dip each fish fillet first into beaten egg mixture, and then into breading mixture. Cover each fish fillet breast well. Place each one on a plate until ready to fry.

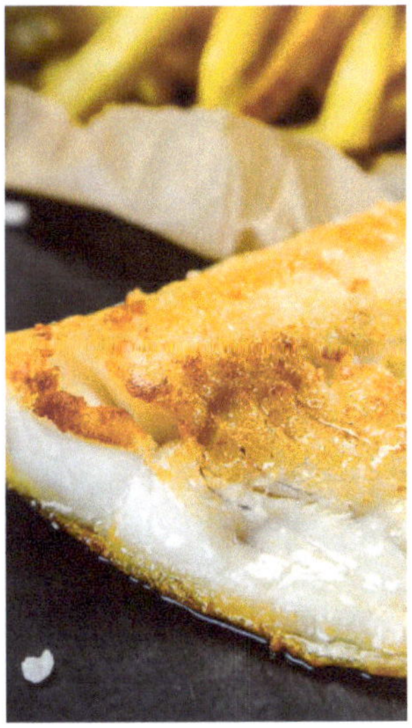

Meanwhile add oil to a large pan and turn on high to bring the oil to frying temperature. Do not overheat oil as it can catch on fire. Be ready with at least some fish fillets to add to the pan. Cook breaded fish fillets on medium high fire and turn them over half way through. Cook until they are golden brown on each side. Remove each fillet from the pan with a slotted spoon and place on plate covered in paper towels to absorb excess oil.

While fillets are frying, prepare tartar sauce. Slowly drizzle and mix olive oil into the Vegenaise. Then slowly add lemon juice and mix. Blend in relish, salt and pepper and serve in ramekins.

Prepare side of spinach or salad by tossing it with parmesan cheese, olive oil, lemon juice, salt and pepper. Serve on side of plate and place fish fillets next to it. Top with a slice of lemon.

Serves 6-8 people ***(Autumn, Winter, Spring)***

Pair with: A side of steaming basmati rice.

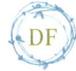

DF GF

Buffalo Lettuce Wraps - Corinna's Creation

This was inspired from a favorite dish in a restaurant nearby that tasted delicious but due to allergens I was not able to enjoy. Instead I put together what I thought would match that flavor and came up with a delicious and crispy recipe.

- 1 cup chopped Vidalia onion
- 1 cup chopped red bell pepper.
- ½ cup finely chopped celery
- 1 cup sliced baby portabella mushrooms
- ¼ cup loosely chopped parsley
- Season Salt to taste
  (mix of salt, paprika, turmeric, garlic & onion powder, cayenne)
- 2 lbs. of buffalo minced meat
- 1 tbsp. rice vinegar
- 8 large washed lettuce leaves

Sauté chopped onion in 2 tbsp. olive oil for about 3 minutes or until onion becomes translucent.

Add chopped red bell pepper and chopped celery into pan and sauté for another 3 minutes.

Add chopped portabella mushrooms, and gently sauté with remaining ingredients. Add parsley and season salt then remove to a side plate.

Use same pan to sauté minced buffalo meat, until well browned. Add a little more seasoned salt to taste and 1 tbsp. rice vinegar. Add sautéed vegetables and mix well.

Take washed lettuce leaves, scoop a generous portion of the meat mixture on them, roll and enjoy.

Serves 4 people ***(Winter, Spring)***

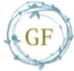

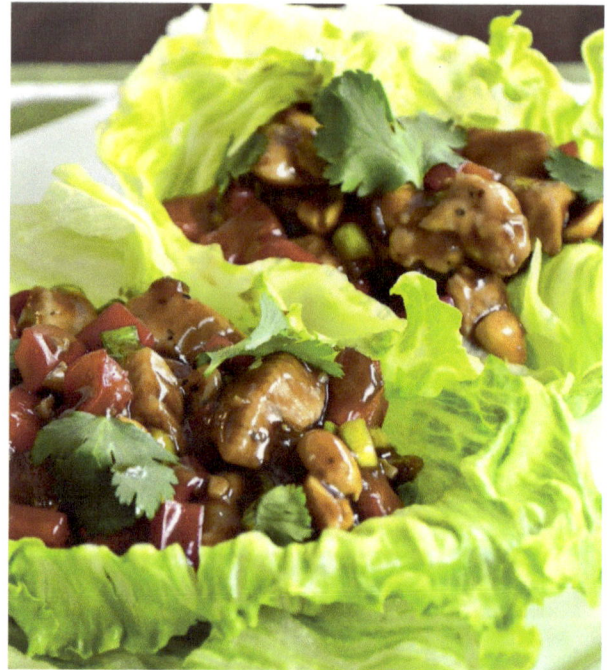

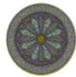

GF

Chicken Breast With Leek, Eggplant & Brown Rice - Corinna's Creation

We love leeks for their sweet and smooth taste and we add them to many of our dishes. This is just one version combined with chicken.

1	large eggplant, peeled and quartered
4	tbsp. olive oil
⅓	cup of water
2	large leeks, including greens, chopped
3	organic boneless chicken breasts, cubed
14	oz. organic chicken broth
4	tbsps. ghee (clarified butter)
1	cup organic brown rice
2	cups water
	Salt & Pepper to taste
1	tsp. Zatar seasoning
	• Avocado slices
	• Lemon wedge
	• Cilantro for garnish

Wash and peel eggplant. Cut in small pieces, set in colander, and dust with salt. Let stand for about 30 minutes to remove bitterness then squeeze excess moisture, rinse well and dry with paper towels. In a medium pot, add ghee and melt over medium high heat. Add rice and sauté for about 5 minutes while mixing constantly. Add 2 cups of water, 1 tsp. salt, mix, cover pot and bring to boil. Once boiling, lower heat to low and cook for about 30-40 minutes.

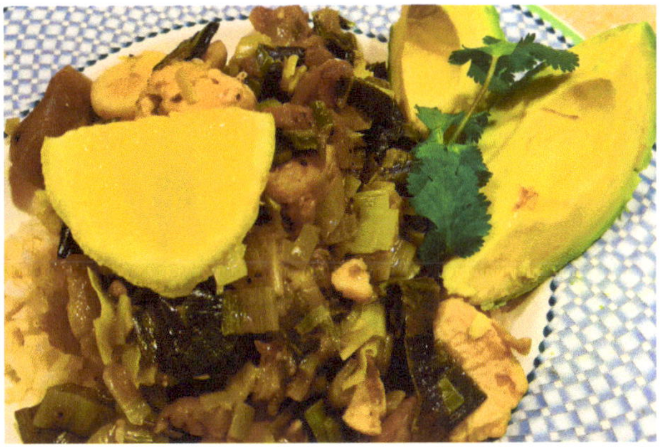

Place eggplant in large pan with 2 tbsp. of olive oil and water and cook over medium/high heat for about 20 minutes or until eggplant looks soft. Add some water if needed. Add leeks and remaining olive oil to the pan and cook until translucent.

In a separate pan, add 2 tbsps. of ghee and cook chicken through until slightly browned, about 10 minutes.

Add chicken to eggplant mix, along with the chicken stock/broth and bring to boil. Season with salt, pepper and Zatar. Lower heat and cook for about 5 minutes to integrate flavors.

Serve over brown rice with a side of avocado slice and lemon wedge.

Perfect for spring and fall.

Serves 6 people *(Spring, Summer)*

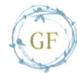

DF GF

From Scratch - Main Dishes

Cailan's Lamb Meatballs

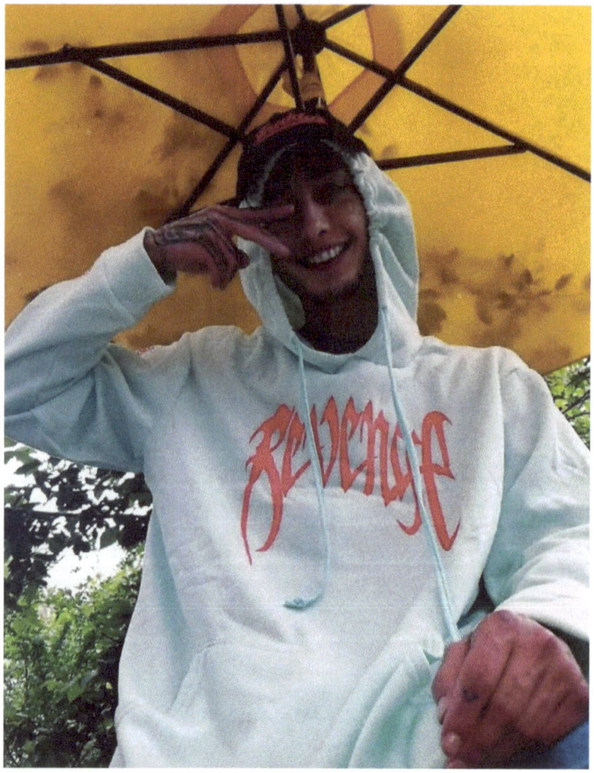

Lamb meatballs were created by my son on one of his lamb meat kicks. He loves to dabble in the kitchen and came up with this recipe out of the blue. Deliciously crispy with a deep delectable taste. Although we do not often eat fried foods, this hit the spot!

- 1 lb. ground lamb
- 1 tsp. sea salt
- 1 tsp. sweet paprika
- ½ tsp. coconut flake powder
- ½ tsp. onion powder
- ½ tsp. garlic powder
- ½ tsp. black pepper
- ¼ tsp. green & red bell pepper powder
- ¼ tsp. dry brown mustard
- ¼ tsp. dry cilantro
- ¼ tsp. celery seeds
- ⅛ tsp. dry thyme
- ⅛ tsp. dry oregano
- ⅛ tsp. dry ginger
- ⅛ tsp. crushed red pepper flakes or cayenne
- ⅛ tsp. lemongrass powder
- • Dash of fennel
- 2 cups flour for coating the meatballs (use Gluten Free flour if preferred)
- 1 cup of half and half (we use almond milk in place of dairy)
- • Grape seed oil for frying

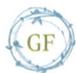

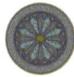

GF DF

Cailan's Lamb Meatballs

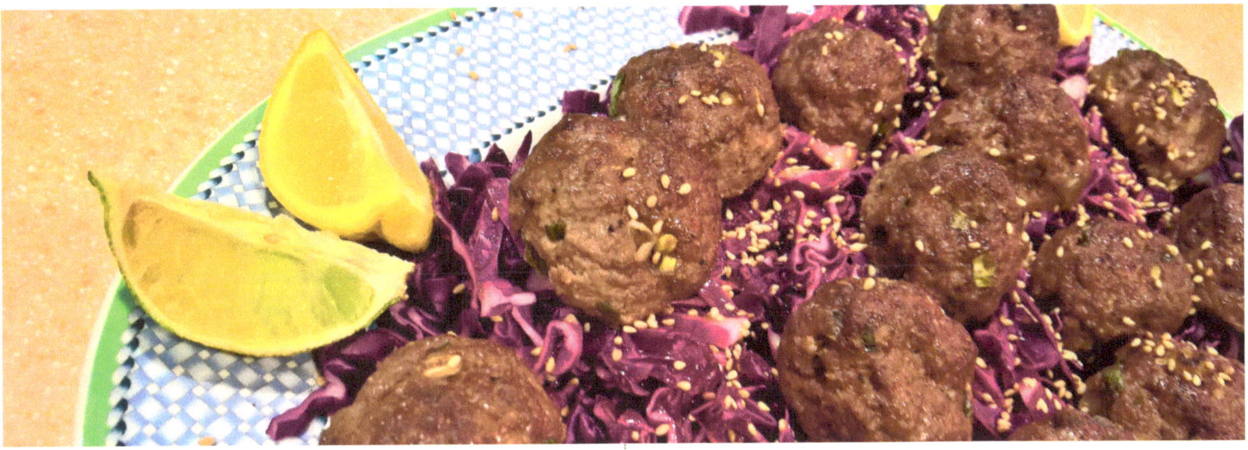

Blend your spices well before mixing them into the flour in a medium low dish. Prepare another shallow dish and fill it with your half and half, buttermilk or a dairy alternative.

From the lamb meat, shape 12 lamb meatballs and place on a tray. Try to shape the balls in similar size to ensure that they cook evenly.

Take your meatballs, one by one, and roll them in the flour/spice mixture until they have a thick coat and it becomes hard to see the meat.

Dip your meatballs into the half and half/buttermilk bowl and then once more transfer it back into the flour and roll them again for a second coat of flour. If you like extra crispy fried food, you can double the dips of the meatballs – half and half/flour and again, half and half/flour.

Once all meatballs have been coated, drop them into a hot fryer until golden brown. For a medium size meatball it takes about 4 minutes to cook well.

If you have doubts, remove a meatball and cut it in half to see if it is cooked fully and safe to eat. If there is no visible red meat, remove the rest of the meatballs and place on a paper towel to soak the extra oil.

Serve with your side dish or a salad and enjoy!

Serves 2-3 people, yields about 10 meatballs
(Autumn, Winter, Spring)

Pair with: a side of green beans & mashed potatoes.

Grilled Lemon Chicken - Corinna's Creation

Lemon is a common ingredient in many of our recipes and for this chicken dish letting it marinate for at least half an hour gives a juicy and rich tasting experience.

2.5 lbs. chicken breasts
Juice of three large lemons
3 tbsp. olive oil
½ tsp. marjoram
1 tsp. salt and a dash of pepper or salt + pepper to taste
eggs, lightly beaten
2 lemons cut in half for the grill

Wash and dry chicken and lay flat in a dish. Poke chicken breasts with a fork all around preparing it for the marinade. Douse breasts with lemon juice and olive oil and sprinkle herbs and seasoning on top on both sides. Let chicken rest and marinate in the fridge for at least half an hour.

Place your marinated chicken breasts on a heated grill and cook for about 7 minutes on each side, depending on thickness of chicken breast. You can brush some of the lemon marinade on the chicken as it cooks to keep it moist.

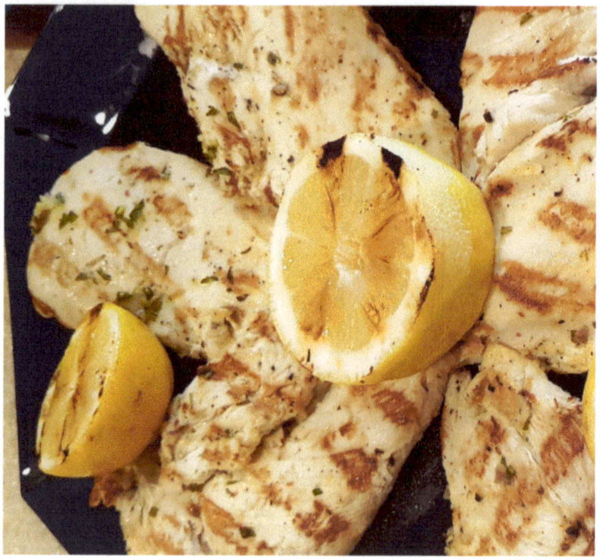

On the side of the grill place your lemon wedges and grill until they have grill marks and are nice and warm. This not only gives the lemon wedges a nice look but it also makes them juicier.

Remove chicken breasts from the grill and onto a platter and let them rest for about 5 minutes before serving. Garnish with lemon wedges.

Serves 6-8 people *(Summer, Autumn, Winter, Spring)*

GF DF

Chicken, Roasted - Kotopoulo ston fourno

Κοτόπουλο στον φούρνο

Oven Roasted Chicken with lemon.

1 5 lb. whole chicken
¼ cup olive oil
2 garlic cloves (minced)
2 lemons, large (juiced)
2 tsps. dried oregano
2 tsps. dried thyme
½ tsp. dry, crushed rosemary
½ tsp. dry marjoram
• Salt + Pepper to taste
10 medium potatoes (cut in wedges)

Wash and dry chicken and place in pan, breast facing down. Preheat oven to 450° F.

Mix spices and pound with mortar and pestle. (Save 1 tbsp. of spices for potatoes.) Rub chicken with 2 tbsps. olive oil and then cover whole chicken with herbs.

Arrange cut up potatoes in the pan around the chicken.

Combine remaining olive oil and 1 tbsp. herbs in a jar with squeezed lemon, salt and pepper and blend well. Pour oil mixture over potatoes and chicken. Place pan in preheated oven, turn temperature down to 375° F and bake for 40 minutes. Baste chicken with juices from pan every 15 minutes and return to oven for another 45 min-

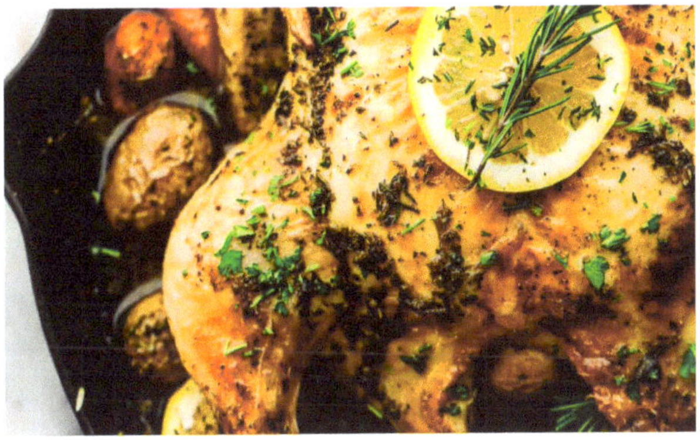

utes or until chicken leg easily pulls off the side. Basting the chicken often will help keep it moist and bake the skin to a golden brown.

Remove chicken from oven and let rest for at least ten minutes to retain its moisture.

If potatoes are not cooked, turn bird over, add water to the pan if needed and roast for another 20 minutes or until potatoes look golden brown and feel soft when poked with a fork.

*If you like carrots, sliced carrots are a nice addition to this dish.

Serves 6-8 people

(Autumn, Winter, Spring)

Pair with: a beautiful tomato and green onion salad with olive oil and red wine vinegar dressing.

DF GF

Chicken Milanese - Breaded Fried Chicken Breast

Κοτόπουλο Μιλανέζ

This meal has a funny story behind it. When I was growing up in Greece, chicken Milanese or otherwise known as Schnitzel, was our family's Saturday meal. This dish was so well liked that we used to have lunch competitions over who would eat the most pieces during the meal.

Now given they were not huge portions, more like small medallion sized cuts of chicken, but even so, the record reached 14 pieces eaten at one sitting by one person! To this day, this is one of our family's favorite dish and for many years now I prepare it with gluten free breadcrumbs, which gives the chicken the same crisp and flavor to it.

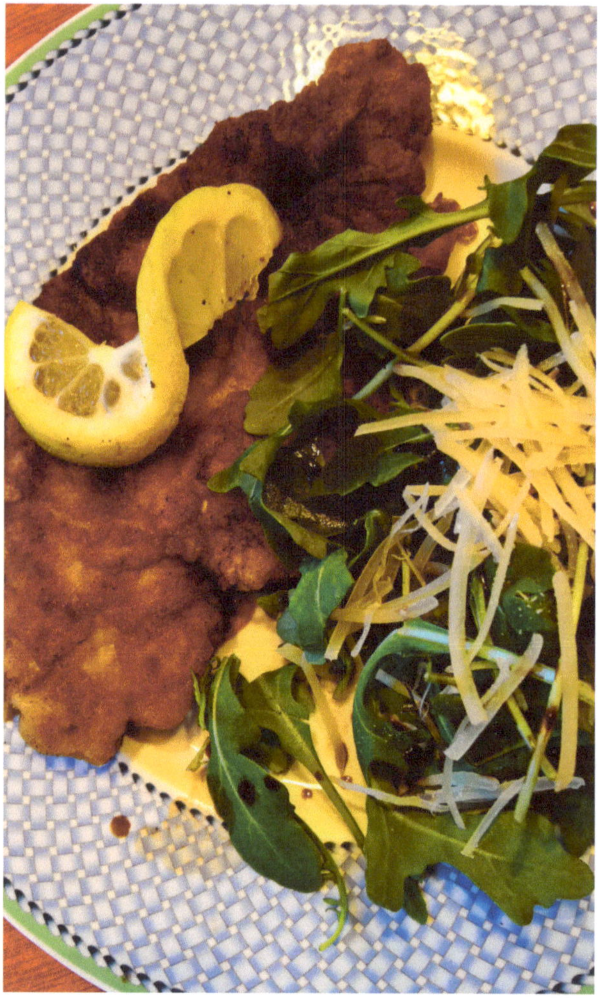

- 2.5 lbs. chicken breast, butterflied & pounded flat
- 4 eggs, lightly beaten
- 2 cups regular or gluten free bread crumbs
- Salt + Pepper to taste
- 1 cup Safflower Oil or other high heat oil
- 1 lemon sliced
- 1 lemon cut in half to squeeze over chicken as needed
- 16 oz. baby arugula
- ⅓ cup shredded parmesan cheese
- 2 tsps. Olive oil
  - Drizzle fresh squeezed lemon juice
  - Salt + Pepper to taste

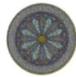

GF DF

Chicken Milanese - Breaded Fried Chicken Breast

Κοτόπουλο Μιλανέζ

Wash and dry chicken, then butterfly breasts or slice each breast in three depending on thickness. Cover chicken slices with cellophane/saran wrap and pound meat with mallet until thin and even. This helps the chicken cook evenly and thoroughly.

Add salt and pepper with breading into a shallow dish and mix. Dip each slice of chicken first into the beaten egg mixture, and then into bread crumbs. Cover each chicken breast really well.

***Optional:** you can dip the chicken into beer first, and then into the bread crumbs, then the egg mixture and then the bread crumbs again for a fuller and puffier tasting chicken breast. Since beer is not gluten free, I have avoided this way for a few years due to our family's allergies. Alternatively to achieve that extra crispy schnitzel taste, dip into the egg, then the breadcrumbs, then the egg again and back into the breading (twice).

Place each one on a plate until ready to fry. Towards the end of breading the chicken, add oil to large pan and turn on high to heat up the oil to frying temperature. Do not overheat oil as it can catch on fire. Be ready with at least some chicken breast to add to the pan.

Continue preparing your chicken breasts until all of the pieces are breaded. Fry chicken pieces in a medium high fire in a light layer of oil and turn breasts over half way through. Generally if the chicken breasts are pounded thin enough, this takes about 3 minutes on each side. Cook until they are golden brown all around.

Remove chicken from fire with a slotted spoon and place on plate covered in paper towels to absorb excess oil.

*Omit parmesan for a dairy free version.

Prepare baby arugula side by tossing it with olive oil, parmesan cheese, lemon juice, salt and pepper. Serve on side of plate and place chicken schnitzel next to it. Top with a slice of lemon.

Serves 6-8 people *(Autumn, Winter, Spring)*

DF GF V

Chickpeas with Leeks

Ρεβύθια με πράσο και άνηθο

A fall Greek dish that is warm an inviting.

- 4 tbsps. olive oil
- 2 cups dry chickpeas (may use canned if pressed for time)
- 4 large leeks, chopped (white and greens)
- 3 cups vegetable broth or
- 2 tbsp. organic vegetable broth concentrate & 3 cups of water
- ⅓ cup fresh squeezed lemon juice (2 large lemons)
- ¼ cup fresh dill, chopped
  - Salt + Pepper to taste

Chickpeas are wonderfully nutritious and make delicious stews and soups. Their shell is a good source of calcium and they provide good fiber, so it is preferable to use them whole. If you are using dry chickpeas, make sure to put them in cold water the night before and allow them to soak overnight. This way they become more easily digestible and cook faster too. Some people will cook them in their original soaked water and others will use fresh. While the soaking water can have a lot of nutrients, if you have digestions problems, it is often better to use fresh water to cook your chickpeas in. I use a pressure cooker to cook mine, but you can just add them to a pot, fill with water and boil until they are soft.

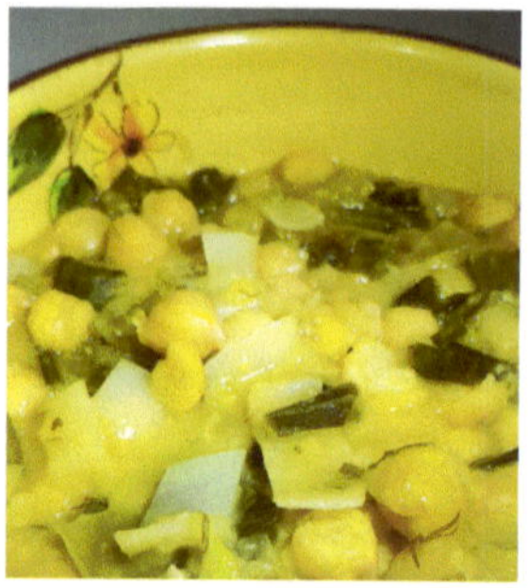

Leeks need to be well washed, as they tend to hold a lot of dirt between the layers. It is easier to slice cross length and wash in between each leaf being careful to not separate them too much before you chop them into round slices.

Once your chickpeas are cooked, in a new pot, add olive oil and chopped leeks and sauté in medium fire until they are translucent and soft – about 10 minutes. Add cooked chickpeas and mix well, sautéing for a few more minutes. Add your vegetable broth or water to cover the mix and bring to a boil. If you are using a vegetable concentrate, first dilute the 2 tablespoons in warm water and then add to the mix with another 3 cups of water to cover the chickpeas.

Add salt and cook for about 15 minutes until the mixture seems thick and ready. Add water during cooking if needed. This dish is usually served more as a thick mixture than a soup, but go with what you like best. At the end add dill, lemon juice and pepper and mix well. Serve warm.

Serves 6 people ***(Autumn, Winter, Spring)***

Pair with: Serve with a slice of feta cheese on the side, as a side dish or eat as a soup.

GF DF

Fish, Grilled, whole

Red snapper, mackerel, swordfish, red mullet and sea bass are some of the fish that Greeks enjoy often. Many times smaller fish comes whole, head and everything, and that is how we grill them. Most of the times when you buy whole fish it will be already cleaned out, but you can always ask for it to be prepped before you buy it.

If you like grilled fish this is one of the easiest ways to prepare them and it is very healthy and filling. Alternatively you can wash them, lightly coat in flour and fry them.

4 small fish of your liking

1 tbsp. olive oil to brush fish before grilling

Ladolemono Sauce

¼ cup olive oil

1 lemon, juiced

- Salt to taste
- Drizzle lemon juice into olive oil while continuously whisking and until well blended. Add salt and serve over fish

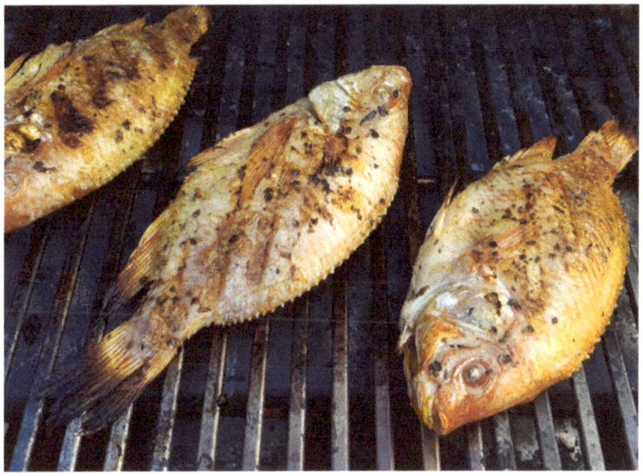

Rinse out your fresh fish and lightly coat with olive oil. Set on a hot grill and cook for about 4 minutes on each side depending on the size of the fish. If the meat flakes easily your fish is ready.

Remove onto a platter and drizzle with "Ladolemono" sauce before serving warm.

Serves 6 people *(Summer)*

Pair with: A simple green salad pairs nicely with the fresh fish.

DF GF

From Scratch - Main Dishes

Keftedes or Kofta

Κεφτέδες

In Greek we call them Kefte or Keftedes for plural, in Lebanese you might find them as Kofta. This rich recipe can be made with beef or a beef and lamb mixture and is amazing on the grill or in the oven. It is similar to the common hamburger except it is loaded with herbs and spices. You can shape the Keftedes into round or oblong pieces and they are delicious either baked or grilled.

- 2 lbs. organic minced beef, or half beef/half lamb
- 1 diced onion
- 3 cloves of minced garlic
- ½ cup of bread crumbs
- 2 tbsps. chopped fresh mint or parsley
- 1 tsp. sea salt
- 1 tsp. sumac (Mediterranean spice blend)
- ½ tsp. black pepper
- ½ tsp. cumin
- ½ tsp. paprika
- ½ tsp. cinnamon (optional)
- ½ tsp. cardamom powdered
- 1 tbsp. olive oil

In a large stainless steel bowl mix beef and all the spices until they are all well blended. Take some of the mix in your hands and roll large meatballs and then shape them into fat cigars. If you will be cooking them in the oven, then shape them all about the same size and place in an oven tray. Cook on convection roast or low broil for about 7 minutes on each side or until meat inside is no longer red. They should be nice and brown when they are ready.

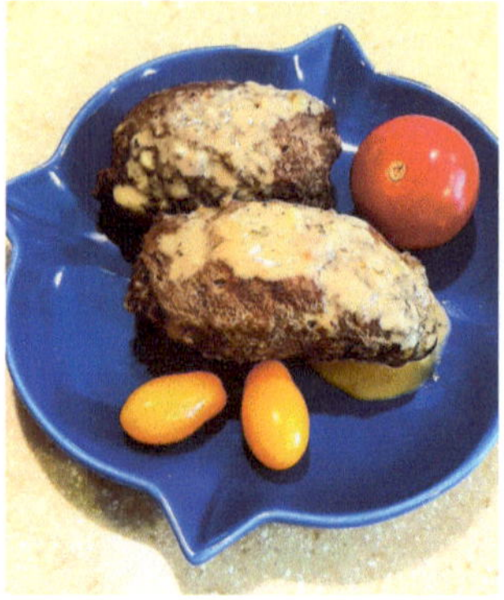

If you would rather grill them you will need to make them a bit thinner. Take a metal skewer and pierce through the Kefte lengthwise and begin squishing the meat on the skewer until it is about 1 inch thick and even all the way across. Put the skewers on the grill and cook for about 3 minutes, making sure to turn them every 30 seconds until they firm up. You need to be vigilant of this process otherwise your kefte might slide off the skewer.

If you like tahini sauce, this dish pairs very well with it. You can find the recipe for Taratur sauce in the Spices, Rubs & Sauces section.

Serve with Taratur sauce.

Serves 4-6 people *(All Seasons)*

*For a gluten free version, use gluten free bread crumbs instead; I prefer the brands that have no added ingredients but just bread crumbs.

GF DF

Lahanodolmades - Rolled Cabbage Leaves Stuffed With Meat, Rice & Spices

Λαχανοντολμάδες

Many Greek dishes involve stuffed or rolled vegetables and these are recipes that seem to go back many generations. Cabbage leaves, grape leaves and fig leaves are some varieties that are often used in the Greek cuisine.

While the smell of steamed cabbage is not the most appetizing, the flavor of the final product is well worth the wait. This is definitely one of our favorites and we make it often during the winter months when cabbage in plentiful.

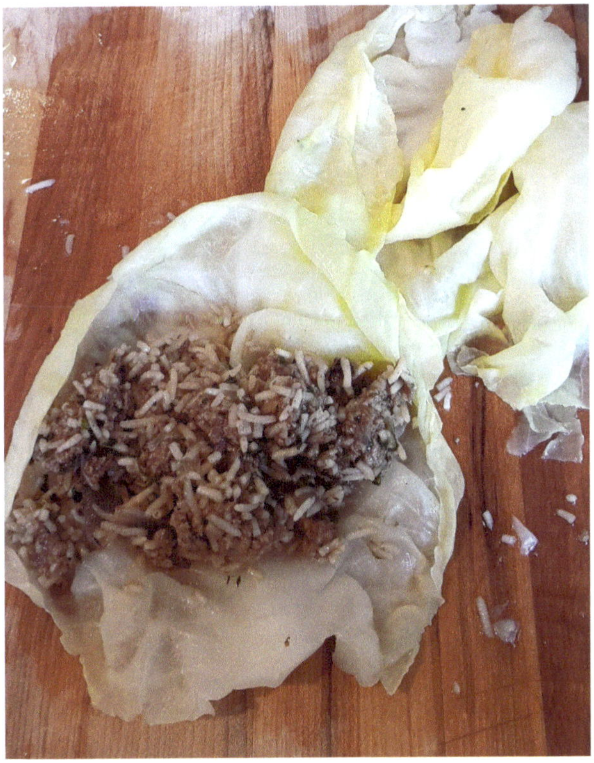

- 1 large green cabbage
- ¼ cup olive oil
- 3 fresh lemons, juiced
- 2-3 eggs, in room temperature

Filling

- 2 tbsps. olive oil
- 1 cup shredded or minced yellow onion
- 1 garlic clove, finely chopped
- ½ cup long grain rice
- ½ lb. organic ground beef
- 1½ cups water
- ¼ cup fresh dill, finely chopped or 1 tsp. dry dill
- ¼ cup fresh parsley, finely chopped or 1 tsp. dry parsley
- ¼ cup fresh mint, finely chopped or 1 tsp. dry mint
- 1 tsp. ground cumin
- • Salt + Pepper to taste
- 1 egg, slightly beaten

Lahanodolmades - Rolled Cabbage Leaves Stuffed With Meat, Rice & Spices

Λαχανοντολμάδες

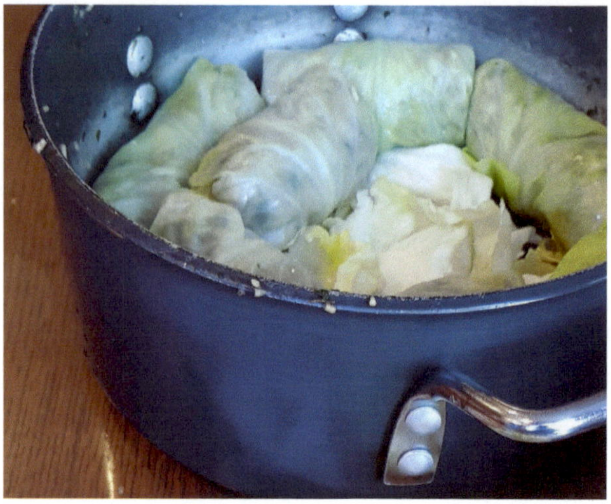

Wash and core cabbage while leaving the vegetable whole and being careful not to damage the leaves in the process. In a large steaming pot add 1 cup of water and place cabbage in pot with the hole facing down. Bring pot to boil, cover and lower temperature to medium allowing the cabbage to slowly steam and the leaves to separate.

This process takes a while, about half an hour; depending on the size of the cabbage. This yields soft large leaves that you can easily roll with. Check the pot to make sure that there is still water and that the leaves are turning a light yellow/green and they become softer. Remove the cabbage from the pot and cool for a while before you begin removing the leaves, one by one, being careful not to tear them.

Alternatively, you may try to separate the leaves while the cabbage is raw, but as they are usually so tightly intertwined, it is easy to damage them in the process.

While the cabbages leaves are steaming, begin preparing the meat filling. In a large heavy skillet add the olive oil and begin sautéing the shredded onions. Once the onions are translucent, add the chopped garlic and give it a minute to soften. Add the rice into the pot and stir while it lightly browns. Add the ground beef and again cook and mix until it is lightly browned as well.

Add ½ cup of water into the filling and mix well. You can now lower the heat and add all the herbs and spices mixing all the while and blending well. Cover the pot and simmer over low heat for about 10-15 minutes, making sure the rice is not fully cooked. You might need to add some more water a little bit at a time, if the rice and meat are sticking. Once the liquid is completely absorbed remove the pot from the fire, uncover and let it cool down.

Now that you have your leaves and filling cooled down you can begin the stuffing and rolling process. First prepare a large soup pot by lining it with a couple of tablespoons of olive oil and any leaves that are too small or torn to be used for rolling. This way you create a layer of cabbage at the bottom of the pot that helps keep the direct heat off your rolls and allows for even cooking.

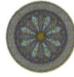

GF DF

Lahanodolmades - Rolled Cabbage Leaves Stuffed With Meat, Rice & Spices

Λαχανοντολμάδες

From your stack of steamed leaves take one leaf at a time, and face the stem your way. Place 2 tbsp. of filling (depending on the size of the leaf it can be more or less) at the bottom side of the cabbage leaf. If your cabbage leaf has a large thick stem, you might want to gently remove that as it will make it hard to roll. With both hands, gently fold each side inward, then roll toward the top of the leaf forming a tight roll. Place each roll into the pot with the seam facing down, so it does not come apart.

Continue this process until you have used all your leaves and have snuggly fit each roll into the pot. You can either place them side by side or form a little snail shape beginning from the center of the pot out. Pour 1 to 1 1/2 cups of water into the pot, enough to rise about 2 inches from the bottom of the pot, the rest of the olive oil and the juice of 1 lemon. Place a serving plate upside down onto the rolled cabbage leaves to keep them from rolling around while cooking. Cover the pot and bring to a gentle boil over medium heat. Then lower your heat and simmer for about 2 hours until the leaves become translucent and very soft. During the cooking process check the level of your water and add ½ a cup at a time if needed.

At the end of the cooking process you need to have about 1 ½ cups of liquid in the pot in order to make the "Avgolemono" sauce before serving the rolls. Once the rolled cabbage leaves are fully cooked, remove from the fire and set aside.

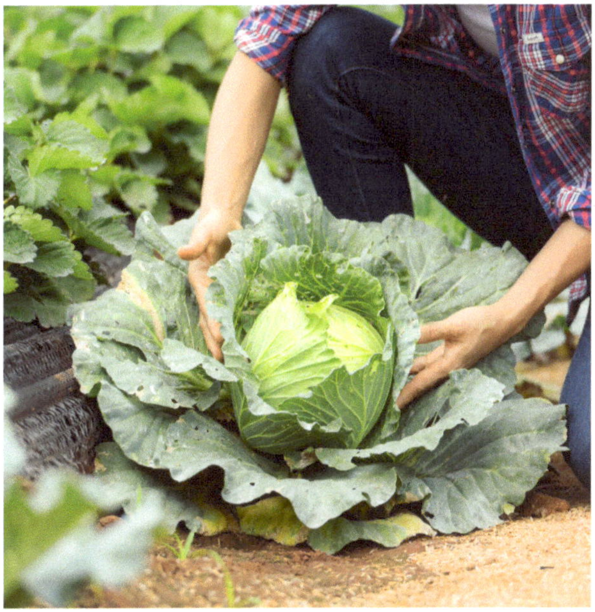

Prepare your Avgolemono sauce (directions under sauces) and gently add back to the pot bringing it all to a slow boil before turning off and removing from the fire.

Serve warm or cold.

Serves 6-8 people

(Autumn, Winter, Spring)

Pair with: This is a very filling meal and we tend to serve it by itself.

Meatballs And Green Beans, Quick & Easy

Κεφτεδάκια

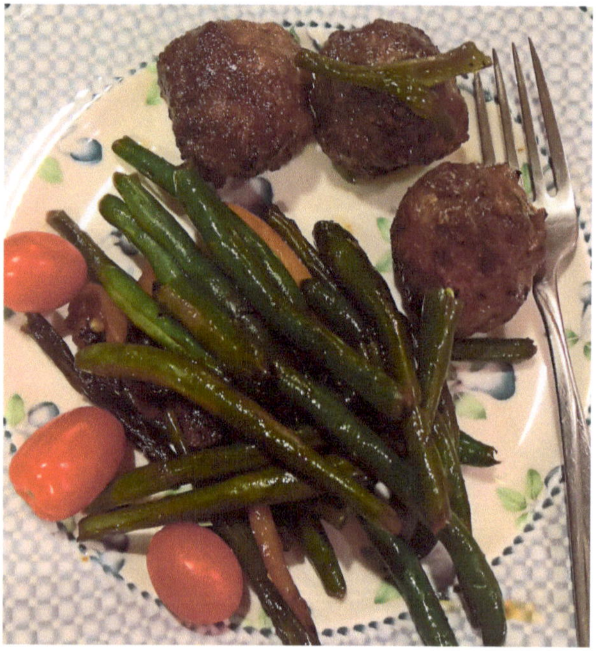

Once again, this is a quick recipe that involves meatballs. Usually a labor of love in the Greek cuisine, as they are normally made with a ton of ingredients and take quite some time to prepare. This is not the case with this simple and fast version of meatballs.

- 2 lbs. organic beef (96% lean)
- ½ cup of bread crumbs
- 1 tbsp. season salt (I prefer Simply Organic brand)
- 1 tbsp. coconut aminos (in the soy section)
- 1 tbsp. dried organic parsley
- 2 tbsps. of water
- ¼ cup gluten free flour for dusting
- 1 tbsp. olive oil

For the side dish:

- 2 tbsps. Greek olive oil
- 1 lb. fresh green beans
- 1 cup red cherry tomatoes sliced in half
- ½ cup slice mini portabella mushrooms
- 2 tbsps. gluten free teriyaki sauce

In a large stainless steel bowl mix beef, bread crumbs, season salt, coconut aminos, parsley and water until they are all well blended. Make small meatballs out of the mixture by taking small chunks of meat and rolling into balls with your hands. Spread flour onto a piece of parchment paper and roll meatballs in it until they are well covered. Spray meatballs with oil and place in large pan in the oven.

Place pan in the oven and cook meatballs under low broil for about 15 minutes, turning them once after 7 minutes. Meatballs should be nicely browned on top.

While the meatballs are cooking, take green beans and wash well in a colander, under running water. Snap off ends and throw into a bowl. Dry beans with a towel

GF DF

Meatballs And Green Beans, Quick & Easy

Κεφτεδάκια

before adding to pan so beans they don't splatter everywhere as they cook. Prepare a large cooking pan with 2 tbsp. of olive oil and set on the stove over high heat.

Add green beans and toss around, mixing the beans constantly until they start wilting, and for about 10 minutes. Cover the pan and let cook for another ten minutes on medium heat. Remove lid and add sliced mushrooms to the pans, while continuing to cook.

After 5 minutes, add teriyaki sauce and continue tossing the beans. Add cherry tomatoes to the pan with the beans and cook for another 5 minutes, until they are sizzled and warmed through.

At the end of the 15 minutes, check on your meatballs to make sure they look nice and brown. Turn the oven off and pull out your pan placing it on a heat proof surface to rest for 5 minutes. Serve meatballs and beans side by side and enjoy.

If you like tahini sauce, this dish pairs very well with it. You can find the recipe for Taratur sauce in the Spices, Rubs & Sauces section.

Serves 4-6 people *(All Seasons)*

* For a gluten free version, use gluten free bread crumbs instead; I prefer the brands that have no added ingredients but just bread crumbs. Also replace dusting flour with a gluten free version.

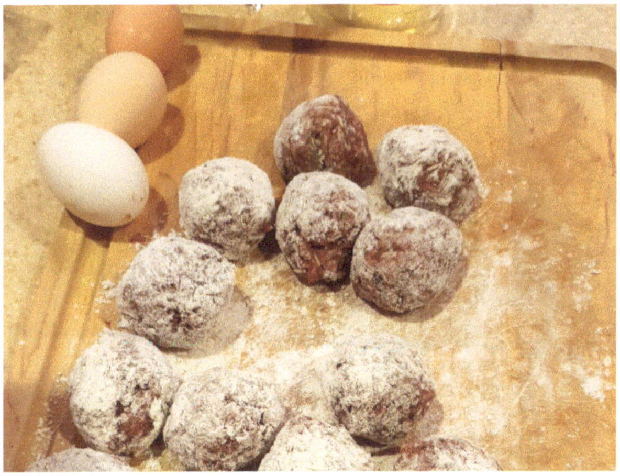

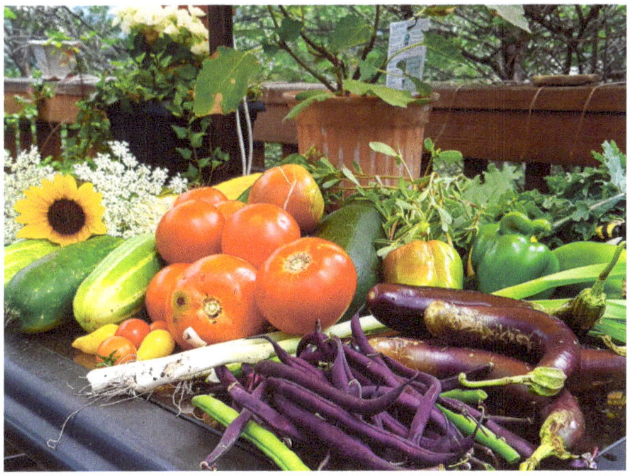

DF GF V

Moroccan Veggie Dish - Another Fall Inspiration

This just came to me one cold autumn day as I was craving the spices and deep flavors of the Moroccan cuisine.

4 tbsps. olive oil
4 large potatoes, thinly sliced in ovals
1 large yellow onion, chopped
4 large squash, thinly sliced in ovals
1 large garlic clove, minced
½ tsp. of garlic powder
(if you don't have fresh)
½ lb. of spinach chopped up fine
1 large green pepper, sliced
1 tsp. of dry turmeric or 1/2 small fresh root grated
• Sea Salt & Pepper to taste
1 tsp. of season salt (mix)
dash of cayenne (optional)
1 organic vegetable bouillon
• Sauté onions and garlic in olive oil until soft and translucent

Add bouillon in pan, smash and let dissolve slowly as you mix it in with the onions and oil.

Add seasonings and dry simmer in pan for a minute or so until you smell the flavors.

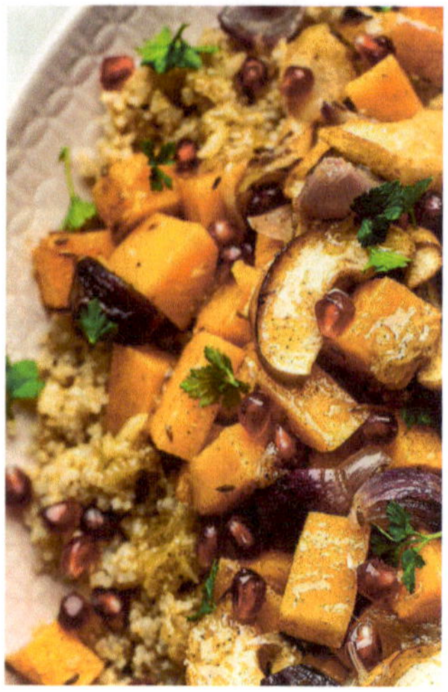

Mix in potatoes and peppers; sauté for 5 mins, then add squash and simmer covered for 15/20 mins. Normally I do not add any water and let the onions and veggies dry simmer in the bouillon and spices. However, if your pan starts to stick, you may add 1/4 cup of water or vegetable stock. The squash will provide the liquid for the dish. Cook until squash and potatoes are soft. Turn off fire, add chopped up spinach and let sit covered for 5 mins.

Mix in spinach and you are ready.

Variations: feel free to use any kind of squash (from zucchini to butternut squash) and add other ingredients such as cooked chickpeas, lentils and other legumes. Just keep in mind that you may need to add more liquid to the cooking process, if you add dryer ingredients.

Serves 6 people ***(Autumn, Winter)***

Pair with: Serve with rice or quinoa as a wholesome vegetarian dish.

DF GF V

Petit Potatoes With Garlic

Healthy, fast, and wholesome.

Perfect for lunch or as a dinner side.

2 cups small white creamer potatoes

2 tbsps. organic Olive Oil

3 garlic slivers, sliced

½ orange bell pepper, sliced

½ red bell pepper, sliced

2 cups cherry tomatoes, sliced

- Salt + Pepper to taste

1/3 cup loosely chopped parsley

Boil small potatoes in a pot until soft, when poked with a fork. In a separate pan, add olive oil and garlic and sauté lightly. Add bell peppers and sauté until soft. Add cherry tomatoes and sizzle till tomatoes become soft, about 2 minutes.

Add boiled potatoes to pan, add season salt or salt and pepper to your liking.

Top with loosely chopped parsley and serve.

*You may add other veggies to the mix according to your liking. Consider sliced button mushrooms, little cauliflower bits or bamboo shoots. Allow some more time for cooking, perhaps add a little water and mix in as above.

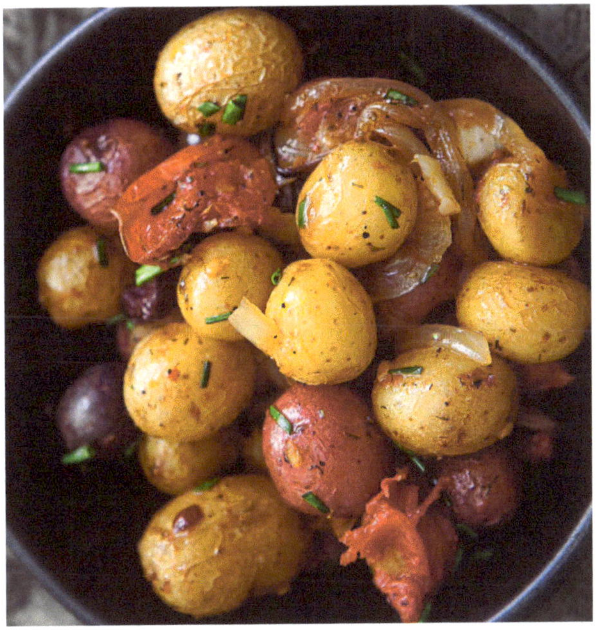

**Tip for slicing large quantities of cherry tomatoes all at once: place tomatoes on a large plate and cover with equal size plate on top. Hold top plate down and insert long bread/slicing knife in between plates, "sawing" through to the other side. Remove top plate and voila! All tomatoes are sliced.

Serves 4 people *(Autumn, Winter)*

Rice Pilaf

This is a speedy version of pilaf as this rice can have an elaborate process. We love to mix pilaf with dishes that have a rich sauce and create a mouthwatering and filling experience. This was one of my favorite side dishes when I was growing up and I remember fondly the addition of cubed carrots and peas in it.

You can choose to add chopped vegetables, as well and mix them in the first five minutes as the rice is cooking. Make sure to have your veggies chopped small so they have ample time to cook by the time the rice is ready.

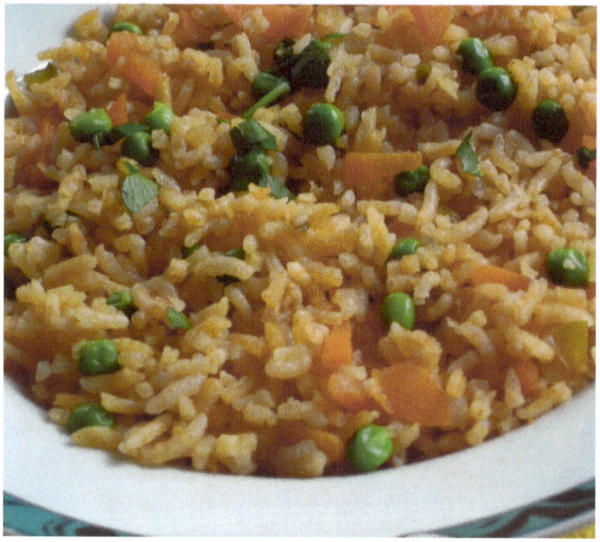

- 2 tbsps. butter
- 1 tbsp. olive oil
- 2 cups Arborio rice
- 2 cups of water
- ½ tsp. season salt
- ½ tsp. turmeric
  - Pepper to taste (optional)
- 2 cups of vegetable broth
- 1 cups of chopped frozen veggies, carrots/peas/corn, rinsed with cold water

Rinse the rice under cold water to remove the starchiness and set aside. In a medium pot, I prefer to use a glass Pyrex, add the butter and olive oil and allow it to melt and blend together. Add the rice and mix continuously over medium high heat, sautéing the rice for three minutes. Pour 2 cups of water into the rice, add salt, pepper and turmeric, stir well and allow it to come to a boil. Lower the fire to a low heat, cover the pot and let cook for about ten minutes. As the rice cooks, the water is absorbed and you can now add the vegetable broth which will give it a smooth taste. If you are adding small chopped vegetables, now is a good time to mix them in. Cook for another ten minutes and then remove pot from fire. Remove the lid and lay a cotton towel over the rice and replace the lid and let it rest for five more minutes.

Serves 6 people ***(All Seasons)***

Pair with: Any saucy main dish.

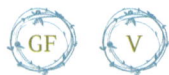

GF DF

Spaghetti With Beef & Mini Bellas - Corinna's Creation

1 package spaghetti (GF version if needed)
1 tbsp. olive oil
2 lbs. organic minced meat
1 cup sliced baby portabella mushrooms
4 cloves roasted garlic
1 organic beef bouillon cube (or 2 cups beef broth)
1 organic mushroom stock cube
• Salt + Pepper to taste
2 cups of water
1 cup of grated parmesan cheese for topping (optional)

Cook pasta according to package directions, adding 1 tbsp. olive oil so they don't stick together. Cover and set aside.

In a separate large and deep pan, sautéed beef until well browned. Pour into a bowl and set aside. In the same skillet add 1 tbsp. olive oil and sauté prepared mushrooms. Once mushroom are starting to soften, add garlic and sauté for another 2 minutes.

Push mushrooms and garlic to the side of the skillet and place 2 bouillon cubes in the center of the pan, mashing and mixing in with the oil. Return cooked beef to the pan and mix with mushrooms. Adds water and blend all ingredients, continuing to cook for another 10 minutes over low/medium heat with the lid on. If you are using

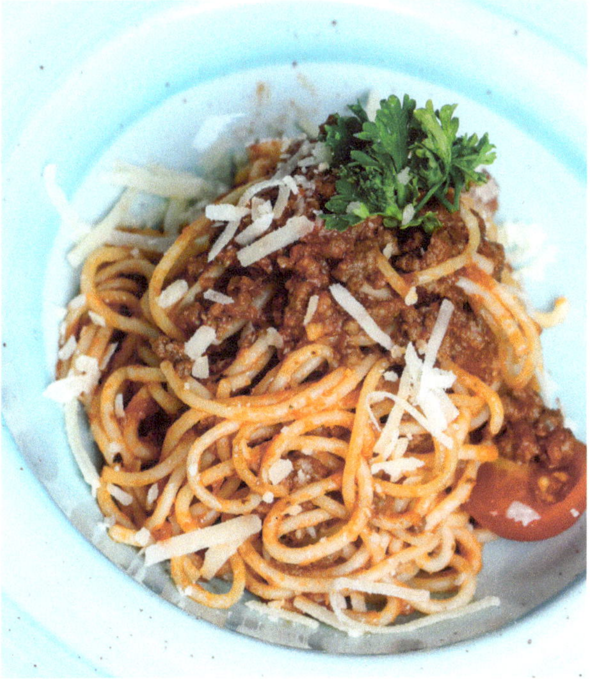

liquid stock/beef broth, just pour the two cups into your skillet, bring to boil and allow to cook with the lid on for about 10 minutes.

Remove lid and cook for another 5 minutes over medium/high heat, scrapping the pan and allowing the broth to thicken. Serve over spaghetti.

Serves 6 people *(All Seasons)*

DF GF

Swordfish Kebab

Wholesome fish on a skewer with tangy spices.

- 2 lbs. thick, fresh swordfish filets cut in chunks
- 1 cup sliced tomatoes or cherry tomatoes
- 1 cup red onions, cut in large chunks
- 1 cup red, green, yellow bell peppers
- 8 laurel leaves
- 2 tbsp. olive oil
- 1 tbsp. dry oregano
- 1 tbsp. dry marjoram
  - Salt + Pepper to taste
- 1 lemon, halved to drizzle on top
  - 6-8 bamboo or metal skewers.
  - Preheat oven to 375° F.

Fresh swordfish is usually available during the winter times and hence this is more of a winter dish. You could prepare this with frozen swordfish but it will not be as juicy. Because swordfish is a very "meaty" fish, it needs lighter spices and veggies to balance its flavor. You can ask your butcher to cut thick fillet slices if possible, which will allow you to cut beautiful 1.5 inch cubes to put on your skewers.

I like to first prepare the fish by patting dry the fillets and removing any excess juices, then cut long strips and cube them. On the side, prepare the vegetables by cutting thick chunks of bell peppers, red onions and tomatoes which will be inserted on the skewers in between the fish pieces to add flavor and color. You can add or substitute other vegetables to your liking such as squash, zucchini, eggplant or mushrooms. Every other piece of fish, I add a laurel leaf, about 2 leaves to each skewer. When you have prepped your fish and veggie pieces, begin assembling your skewers on bamboo sticks. It is helpful to soak the bamboo sticks in water for about 10-20 minutes before using them, that way they will not catch on fire when broiling. You can also opt for metal skewers.

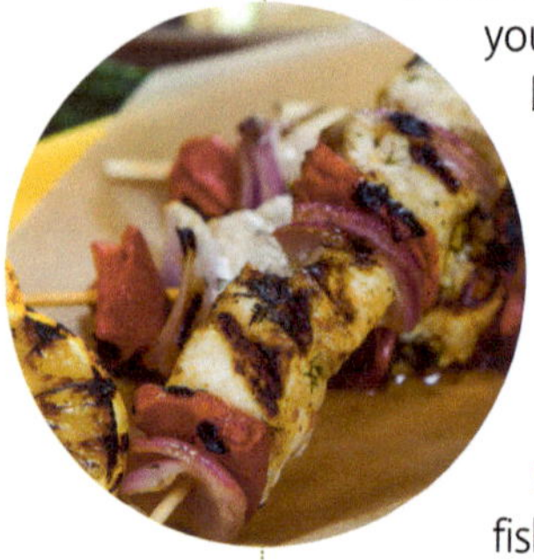

Begin assembling each skewer adding enough fish and veggies for one serving, usually 5-6 cubes of fish interspersed with onions, peppers and tomatoes. Place each skewer in a long enough pan, drizzle with olive oil, and sprinkle herbs and spices uniformly on each side. Insert tray/pan in oven and cook for about ten minutes on each side, top and bottom, until fish looks white and vegetables have become softened.

Change cooking to broil for a couple of minutes in the end to crisp the veggies and add that grilled look to your skewers. Do not overcook or the fish will dry out. Serve immediately with some squeezed lemon on top, over a bed of rice or with a side salad.

Serves 6-8 people ***(Winter, Spring)***

Pair with: steaming basmati rice.

GF DF

Veal, "Reddened"

A hearty dish with braised veal in tomato sauce, perfect for colder months. Beef or lamb may be substituted.

- 6 tbsps. olive oil
- 1 large yellow onion, finely chopped
- 3 large garlic cloves, minced
- ½ cup red wine
- 1 tbsp. tomato paste
- 2 lbs. of stew beef, or veal pieces
- 2 cups of chopped fresh tomatoes or 1 14 oz. can
- 2 tsps. Sea Salt
- • Pepper to taste
- 2 bay/laurel leaves
- 3 dry whole cloves
- 6 cups of water

Sauté beef or veal in a heavy pot (cast iron works great), until beef is well browned. Removed meat into a side bowl for now and add onions and garlic in olive oil sautéing until soft and translucent.

Meanwhile, add tomato paste into ½ cup of wine and mix well to dissolve. As the meat and onions cook for about four minutes, add fresh tomatoes and cook for a few minutes until they dissolve while stirring with a wooden spoon. Add the wine into the pot, as well as salt and pepper, bay leaf and clove and stir well.

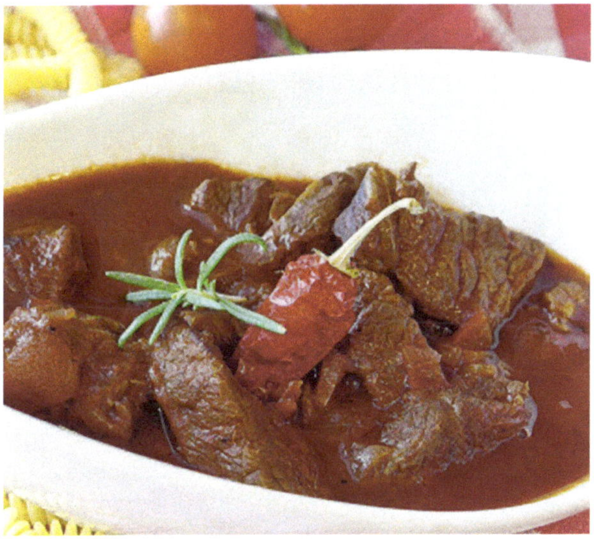

At this point you may add some water, ½ cup or so, turn up the heat to high and bring it to a boil. Continue to add remaining water, a little bit at a time, bringing to boil each time in order to allow sauce to blend well together.

Cover and reduce heat to medium letting it cook for at least two hours. Occasionally, lift the lid and test the doneness of meat and thickness of sauce.

Serves 6 people ***(Autumn, Winter)***

Pair with: Serve with white rice or oven roasted potatoes or even French fries for a hearty meal.

Dolmadakia Yialantzi

Ντολμαδάκια Γιαλαντζί

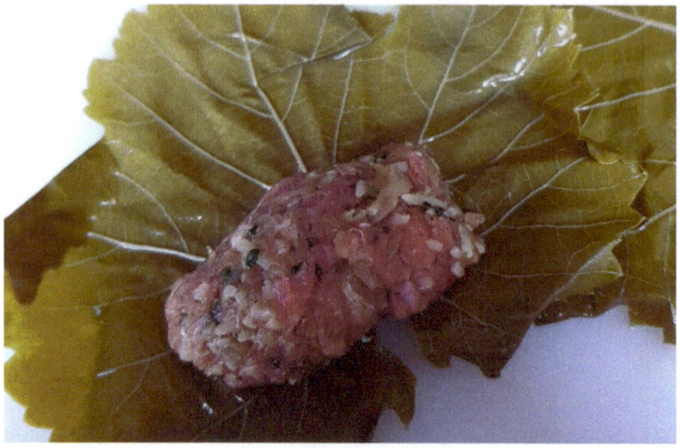

This food is a favorite for the whole family. Dolmadakia can be served as an appetizer or as a main meal, especially if you add meat to it. It is a process that is a bit tedious but the end result is worth the labor. When we make these we usually roll at least a hundred of them, and believe me they go fast! Traditionally, I had only tasted these with rice and herbs, but there are variations out there that add different herbs, lentils, and even minced meat.

- 50 fresh or brined grape leaves in a jar
- 8 cups of hot water
- 4 tbsps. Olive oil
- 2 large red onions, finely chopped or grated
- 1 bunch spring onions, finely chopped
- 4 garlic cloves
- 1 cup long grain rice
- 2 medium soft tomatoes, chopped
- ¾ cup fresh parsley, chopped
- ¼ cup fresh mint chopped, *or*
- 1 tsp. dry mint
- 3 tbsps. fresh dill, finely chopped *or*
- 1 tsp. dry dill
- 1 tsp. ground cumin
- Salt + pepper to taste
- 2 cups of boiling water
- 2 tbsps. Olive oil
- 2 lemons, juiced

Fresh grape leaves need some prep work before you can roll them. First off, if you have your own vines, make sure to pick the freshest and softest leaves. You also want to make sure they are large enough to fit enough of the stuffing when you roll them. Generally if they are about the size of your hand, they will be big enough. Boil 8 cups of water, remove pot from fire, and gently submerge the fresh leaves for about 4 minutes. Remove leaves carefully from the pot with a slotted spoon and gently rinse in cool water in a colander and allow to drain.

If you are using store bought leaves, usually packed in brine in a glass jar, remove leaves carefully from the jar before rinsing several times in a colander. This is tricky at

DF GF V

Dolmadakia Yialantzi

Ντολμαδάκια Γιαλαντζί

times as the leaves seem to puff up once in the jar and they become more difficult to remove. I often need to use a skinny wooden spoon to coax them out without ripping them.

In a large pot, heat the olive oil and sauté the red and green onions until they are translucent. Add garlic and sauté a little longer while continuously mixing. Add the rice in the pot, mix to coat well with oil and cook just enough to slightly soften, about 5 minutes. Add the tomatoes and gently mix. Now mix in the herbs, parsley, mint and dill, salt and pepper and remove from heat and let cool.

Take the rinsed leaves and separate any small, torn or uneven leaves from the lot. Use these to line the bottom of your pot. This will help your rolls cook evenly. Take one leaf at a time, rough side up, lay on a cutting board and snip off the hard edge of the stem. Place about 1 teaspoon (depending on the size of the leaf) of cooled mixture in the middle of the leaf towards the bottom and begin rolling from the bottom. Then fold in the left and right sides of the leaf and then roll up tightly forming the shape of a small cigar. Make sure all stuffing is tucked into the leaf.

Then place the roll seam down into the pot. One by one start stacking them tightly next to each other into the pot until you fill the first layer. Then continue on with the second layers and so on until your leaves and your stuffing is finished. Pour the boiling water, 2 tablespoons of olive oil and the squeezed lemon over the rolled Dolmadakia and cover with an inverted plate to keep in place. Simmer gently for 45 minutes to an hour until the rice is cooked and the leaves are tender.

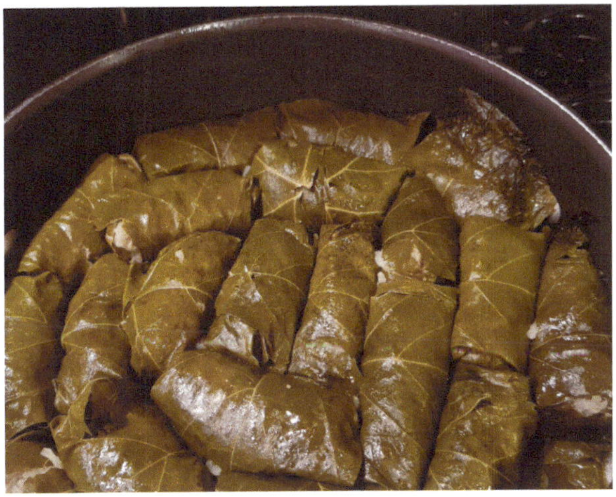

P.S. You can add other ingredients to the mix as well depending on your preference. Some other ingredients that I have tried at times are fennel, minced beef or a mixture of lamb and beef. You can even add cooked legumes in the mix such as lentils for a hearty vegetarian meal.

Tzatziki sauce is a great accompaniment to stuffed grape leaves.

Serves 5 people ***(All Seasons)***

6

Sweet & Tangy Desserts

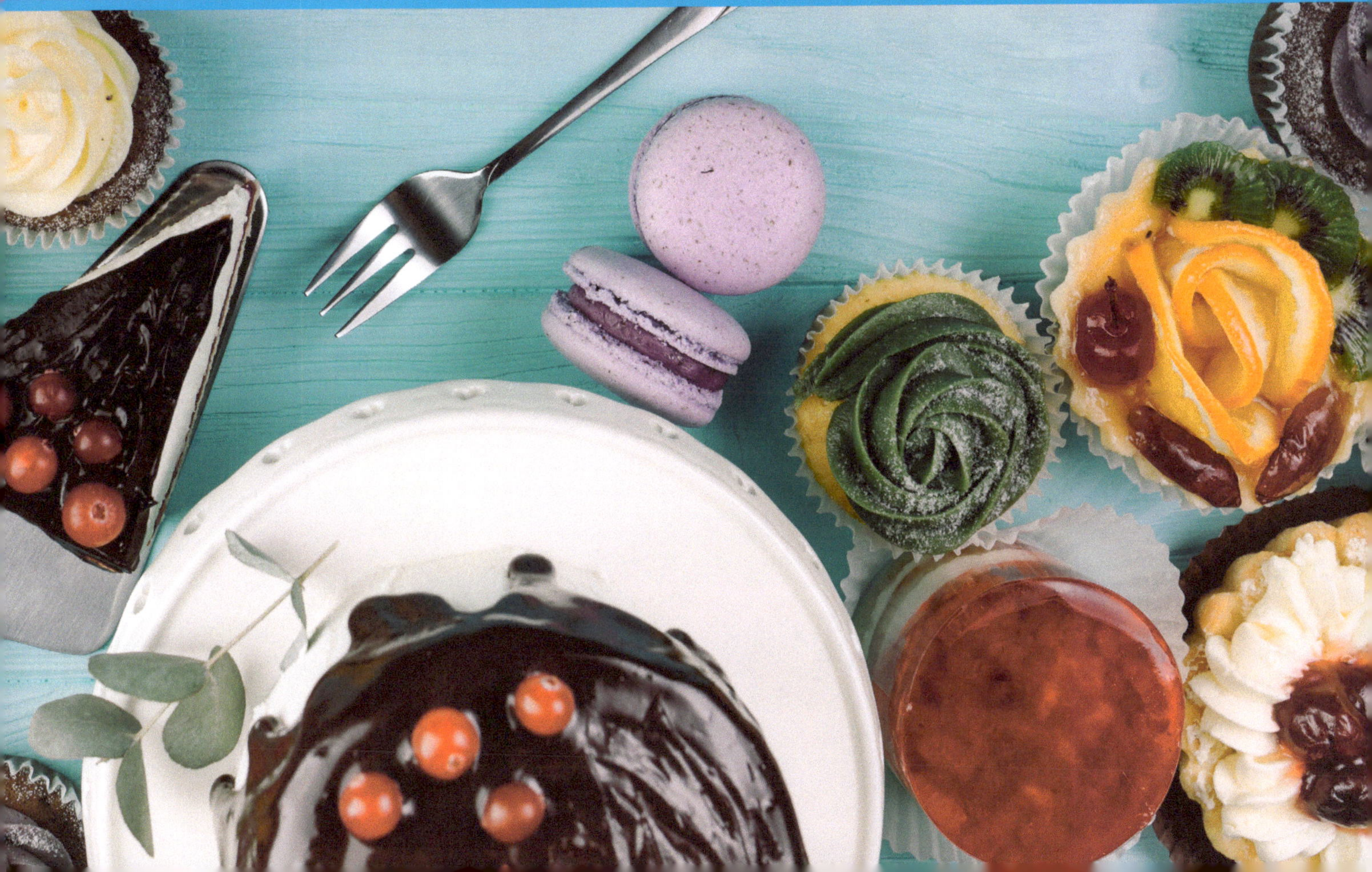

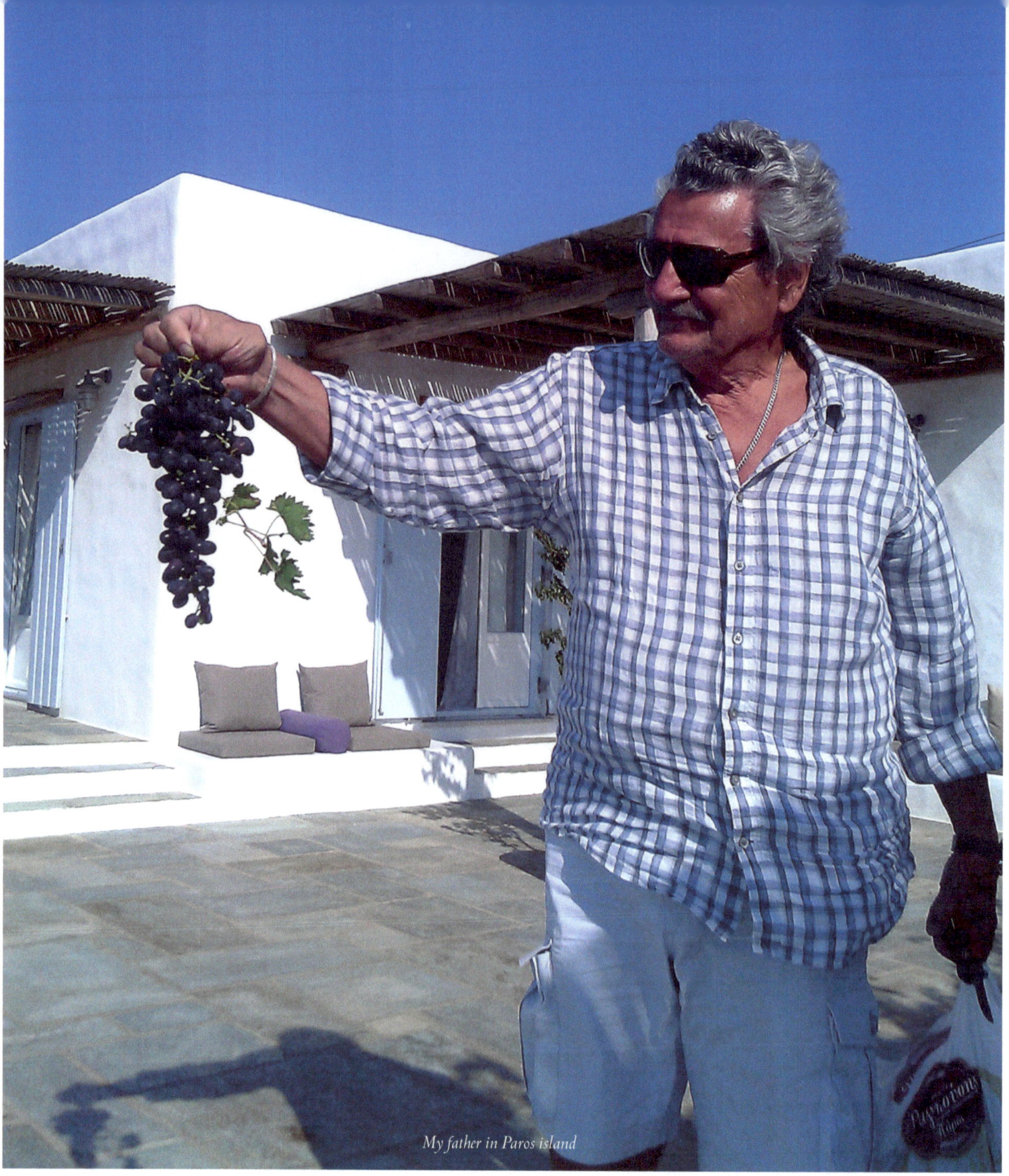

My father in Paros island

Fruit

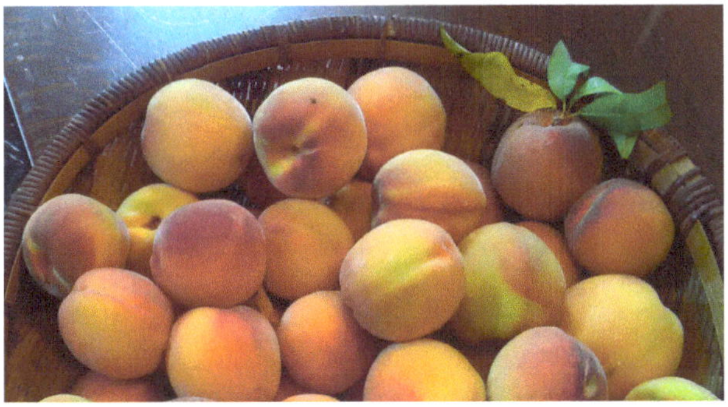

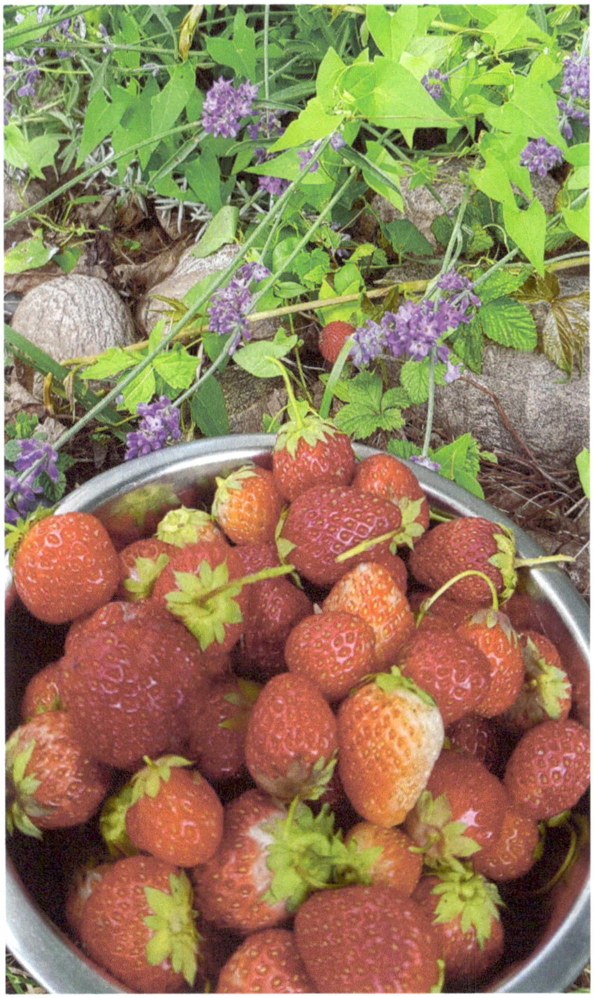

Fresh Fruit is nature's tastiest desert.

Consider ending your meal with some sweet strawberries sprinkled with fresh lemon juice, some cut up melon, a bunch of grapes or even a fruit salad mixed with a bit of orange juice and honey.

Not only is fruit a healthy addition to your diet but fruit also contain good enzymes that help you digest your food. Spiced Apple Slices is a great ending to your meal – you can find this recipe further out in the book.

During the summer months, I go out to the garden early in the morning – the best time to pick fruit and herbs –and pick berries, apples, peaches, plums and whatever else happens to be in season.

And if you have an abundance of fruit consider even making smoothies, fruit juice, a pie, jam and other delicious treats for you and your family.

DF GF V

Sweet & Tangy

Banana Bread - Warm & Gooey

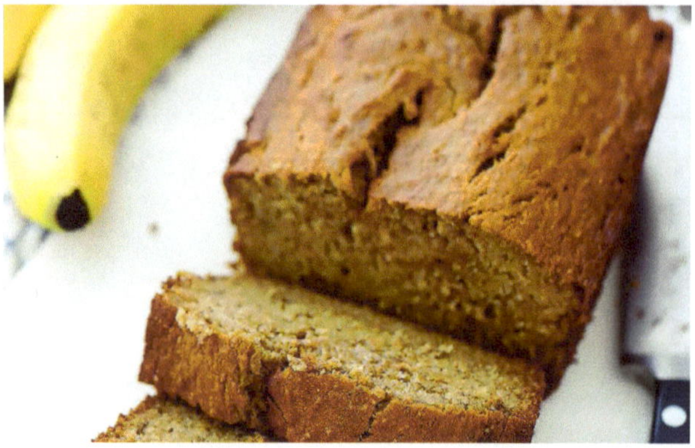

So, I am sure other families experience this as well... you buy a bunch of bananas and bring it home, and before you know it they are all gone. Kid runs into the kitchen and asks if there are more bananas – sorry! At your next trip to the store you buy more bananas to replenish the stash, and lo and behold, they just sit there in the fruit bowl until they become soft and gooey and no one wants them! Enter the trusted banana bread recipe that everyone loves.

- ¾ cups organic raw sugar
- ¼ cup butter, softened or dairy alternative
- 2 medium bananas, mashed with a fork
- 2 tsp. lemon juice
- ⅓ cup of milk
- 2 eggs, beaten
- 1 ½ cups all-purpose or gluten free flour (Bob's Red Mill works well for GF)
- 1 tsp. baking soda (if in high altitude reduce baking soda to ½ tsp)
- ½ tsp. baking powder
- ½ cup chopped walnuts (optional)

Grease a 9x5x3 inch loaf pan and set aside. This mixture can also be poured into a lined muffin pan to make individual breakfast servings instead.

In a food processor cream together butter and sugar until white and blended. Mix in slowly mashed bananas, then lemon juice. If you like sweets, well ripened bananas will work best. Add milk and eggs. Slowly sift in flour, baking soda and baking powder. Blend mixture well in slow setting. Stir in nuts, if using, and pour into prepared pan. (Alternatively use dairy free options mentioned in the introduction).

Convection bake at 325° F for about 40 minutes. For the gluten free version, lower the temperature after 25 minutes to 300° F and bake another 7-10 minutes. Use a toothpick to test readiness. Remove from oven and let rest at least five minutes before turning upside down and serving on a plate.

*For a dairy free version use vegetable shortening and almond milk instead.

Serves 4 people ***(All Seasons)***

Sweet & Tangy

DF GF V

Chocolate Muffins - Gluten Free Version

These ingredients sound funky together, but I promise you these cupcakes are delicious. They were always a hit with kids coming in and out of the house and school functions. They are so much healthier than many versions and gluten free!

- 1 cup gluten free baking mix
- 1 cup Dutch-process cocoa
- 1½ tsp. guar gum
- 1 tsp. xanthan gum
- ¼ tsp. sea salt
- 1 cup wild flower raw honey
- 1 cup milk
- 2 eggs, slightly beaten
- 1½ tsp. liquid vanilla
- ¼ cup olive oil
- 1 tsp. lemon juice

In a large blender bowl stir together dry ingredients then slowly add honey and set aside.

In another medium bowl mix together beaten eggs, milk, vanilla and lemon juice. Whip mixture until blended. In dry mixture bowl slowly add oil, and then add liquids to it while mixing on low speed until ingredients are mixed. Continue to mix for about a minute on medium speed, until blend is smooth. You can also mix ingredients by hand if you wish for a chunkier taste.

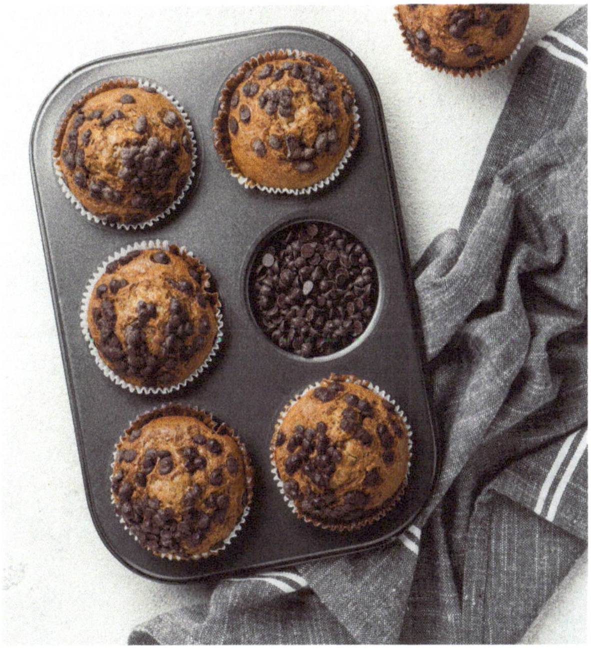

Meanwhile, oil a cupcake pan or use cupcake liners to prepare your pan. Pour mix into cupcake pan, about 2/3 of the way and bake at 375° F for 20 minutes or until toothpick comes out clean.

Let stand to cool a little before removing from pan.

Serves 12 people ***(All Seasons)***

Pair with: Top with whipped cream or icing/topping of your choice.

GF V

Créme Caramel - Greek Style Créme Caramel Pudding

Κρέμα Καραμέλ

This desert is a sweet memory from my childhood. I remember spending so much time as a young child trying to perfect the ratio of caramel to pudding. It was one of my addictions growing up and not an easy desert to master when you are 9 years old. None the less, trying was half the fun. I remember eating the crème caramel while it was still warm in the ramekin. Oh, what a mouthful!

For the Caramel

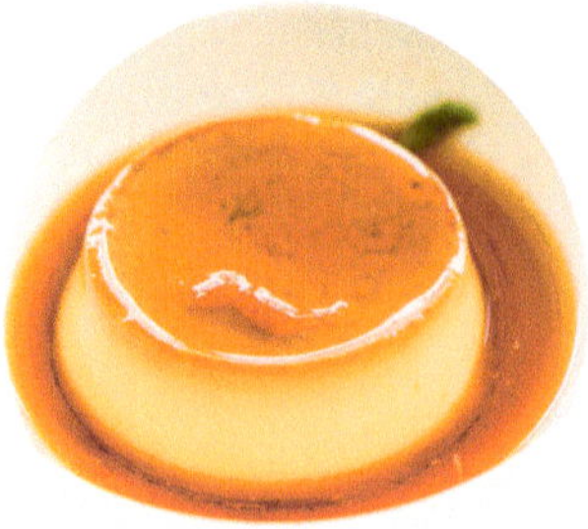

- 1 cup granulated sugar
- ½ cup water

For the crème

- 1 cup milk
- 4 eggs
- 1 cup heavy cream
- 1 tsp. vanilla extract
  - Preheat oven to/ 325° F.

Prepare 6-8 ramekins or foil disposable cups. In a medium-sized pot combine sugar and water over medium heat. Bring to a boil, occasionally swirling the pot, until it becomes an amber color. Once ready, carefully pour caramel into ramekins/cups. Let the caramel sit while you prepare the crème. In the same pot, pour in milk, cream and simmer on low heat.

Do not boil. You should be able to test the temperature with your finger without getting burned. Whisk mixture to blend well and absorb any extra caramel on the sides of the pot. Set pot aside. Meanwhile gently whisk the eggs in a separate bowl and add the vanilla extract. Very slowly drizzle in milk mixture into mixed eggs, while continuously gently whisking keeping a smooth but moving motion. Make sure there is no egg chunks in the mixture and that everything is well blended. If need be, use a very fine sieve like a "chinois" to pass the mixture through. Slowly pour crème mixture into ramekins to equally fill each one almost to the top.

Once your ramekins are full, take a deep baking pan, fill it with warm up to the middle and place the ramekins inside the water. Cover ramekins with foil so they will not burn on top and bake in the preheated oven for about an hour until crème has set. Insert a toothpick in the center of a ramekin to test; if it comes out clean, it is ready. When ready, take each ramekin out of the oven, let cool completely and then refrigerate for 24 hours. You may also serve the crème caramel warm out of the ramekin, if you prefer.

To remove from ramekin after 24 hours, take out of the fridge and immerse in hot water for a few minutes until the crème caramel separates from the sides. You may need to help it by gently running a knife around the edges. Place small plate on top of ramekin and swiftly turn it upside down to release crème caramel onto the plate. Make sure to allow enough time in the hot water as you want the caramel on the bottom of the ramekin to warm up and drip over your crème as you reverse it onto the plate.

Serves 6-8 people *(All Seasons)*

DF GF V

Gluten Free Brownies - Soft & Gooey

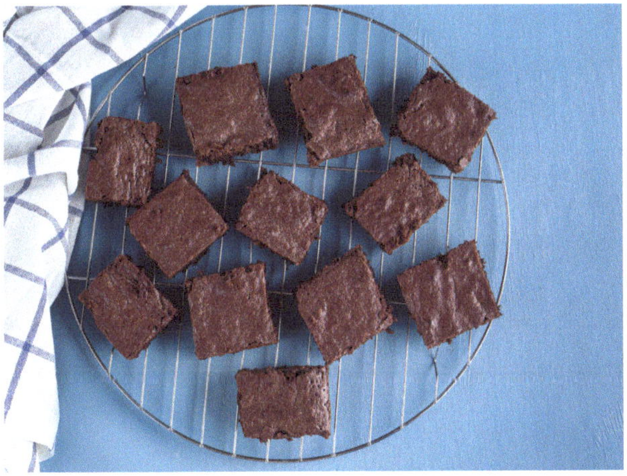

Ok, while brownies are not a Mediterranean recipe, a lot of us may enjoy a nice, chocolatey treat once in a while. While keeping your ingredients fresh and sugar to a minimum in your diet helps you stay healthy and toned, a sweet treat once in a while is essential to supporting the mood and tickling your senses. Fresh, organic cocoa powder is filled with antioxidants. Alternative flours are a staple in our pantry, so if you strive to cook gluten free consider always having these on hand.

Flour blend

- ½ cup brown rice flour
- ½ cup white rice flour
- ½ cup tapioca starch
- ½ cup potato starch

  Or you may substitute the above with 2 cups of your favorite GF flour mixture in the market.

- 2 tbsps. cocoa powder
- ½ -3/4 cup raw sugar (some like it sweeter)
- ¼ cup brown sugar
- ¾ cup gluten free chocolate chips or chunks
- ½ tsp. sea salt
- ½ tsp. xanthan gum
- ½ tsp. baking soda
- ½ cup oil (olive oil is ok and makes for a rich taste)
- 1 large egg, mixed
- ¼ cup water

Grease a 9x9 inch pan and set aside. This mixture can also be poured into a lined muffin pan to make individual servings instead. Mix all ingredients in a bowl with a fork. (Omit egg if needed and add a tsp of oil.) Batter will be thick but do not over mix. Pour into pan and convection bake at 350° F for about 20 minutes until toothpick inserted comes out mostly clean. Remove from oven and let rest at least five minutes before cutting into squares. Serve warm or cold.

Serves 6-12 people *(All Seasons)*

GF V

Rizogalo – Greek Rice Pudding Desert

Ρυζόγαλο

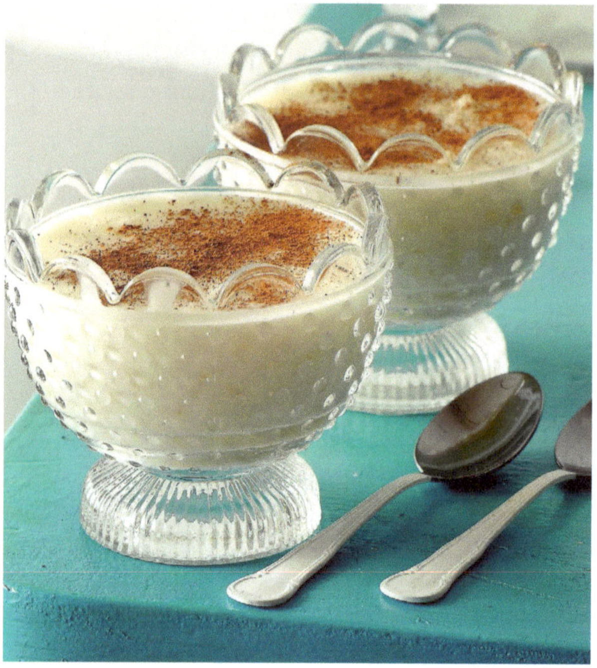

Ah, another one of those deserts that fills your mouth with its creamy warm texture. Rice pudding is very easy to make, although it does take a bit of time. I often enjoy flavoring my pudding with some fresh lavender from the garden. It gives is a gentle underlying taste that brings memories of walking in summer lavender fields. If you want to try that, just take about 1 tablespoon of lavender flowers, wrap them in cheesecloth and let them cook with the rice for 1 hour.

- 1 cup long grain rice
- 6 cups whole milk
- 1 tsps. of butter
- ¾ cups of raw sugar
- 1 cinnamon stick for flavor
- ½ tsp. finely ground Lemon zest
- 1 tsp. vanilla extract
- 2 egg yolks at room temperature

In a medium-sized pot combine milk, rice, sugar and butter and place on low heat.

Simmer for 1 hour allowing the sugar and milk to become thick and the rice to gain size.

Add cinnamon stick half way through.

After 1 ½ hours remove from heat, add lemon zest, and discard cinnamon or lavender. Stir in vanilla. On a side dish beat egg yolks until creamy. Slowly add a little pudding at a time to beaten eggs, and then pour mixture back into main pot and mix altogether.

Let stand to cool in serving containers of your choice and sprinkle with nutmeg or cinnamon. May be served warm or cold.

Serves 10-12 people *(All Seasons)*

Pair with: Light and delicious, pairs well with a lot of dishes.

Sweet & Tangy

DF GF V

Spiced Apple Slices

A quick and easy sweet & tangy taste to clear your palate after a meal.

Honey is a great way to sweeten things and in Greece we use it a lot as a means to prepare simple but delicious deserts after a meal. Local honey is also a great way to keep your allergies in check. Bees that harvest pollen from wildflowers in your area make a special honey that can help your immune system stand up to seasonal allergies.

- 2 granny smith apples
- ⅓ cup freshly squeezed lemon juice
- 2 tbsp. raw honey
- ½ tsp. cinnamon

In this simple but delicious recipe, all you need to do is cut a couple of green granny smith apples into thin slices, arrange in a plate and sprinkle with lemon, honey and cinnamon. Voila!

Serves 6-8 people ***(Autumn, Winter, Spring)***

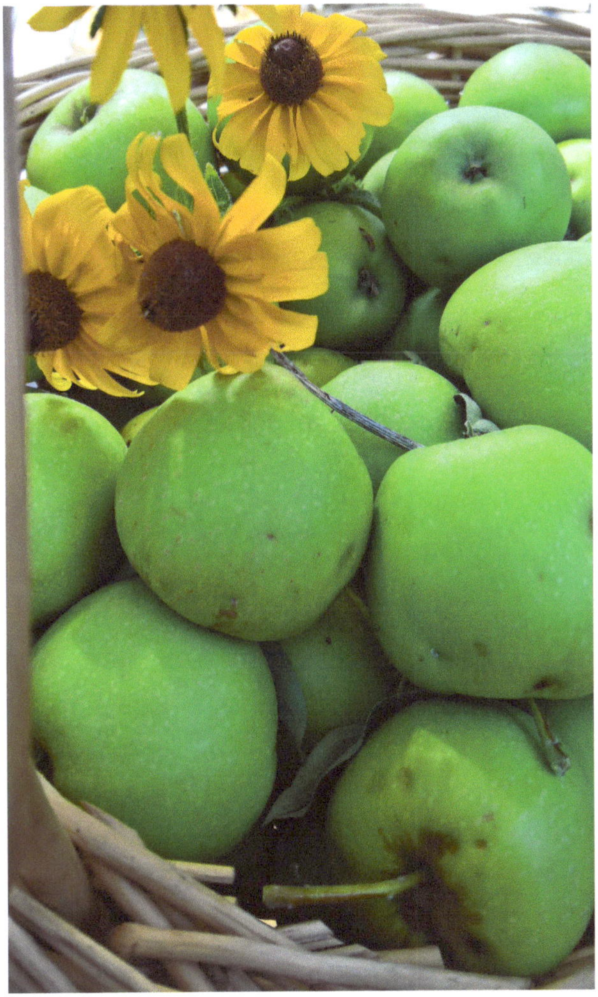

DF GF V

Sweet & Tangy

Sweet Walnuts

Καρύδια με μέλι

Simple & Delicious.

1 cup raw organic walnut halves or pieces
4 tsp wild flower/thyme Raw honey
- Optional: dash of cinnamon

Simply serve walnuts in individual bowls or ramekins, top with honey and cinnamon. A delicious, healthy dessert in minutes.

Serves 4 people *(All Seasons)*

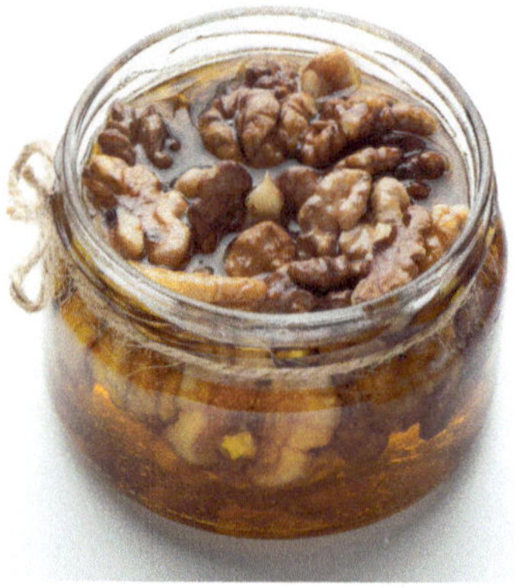

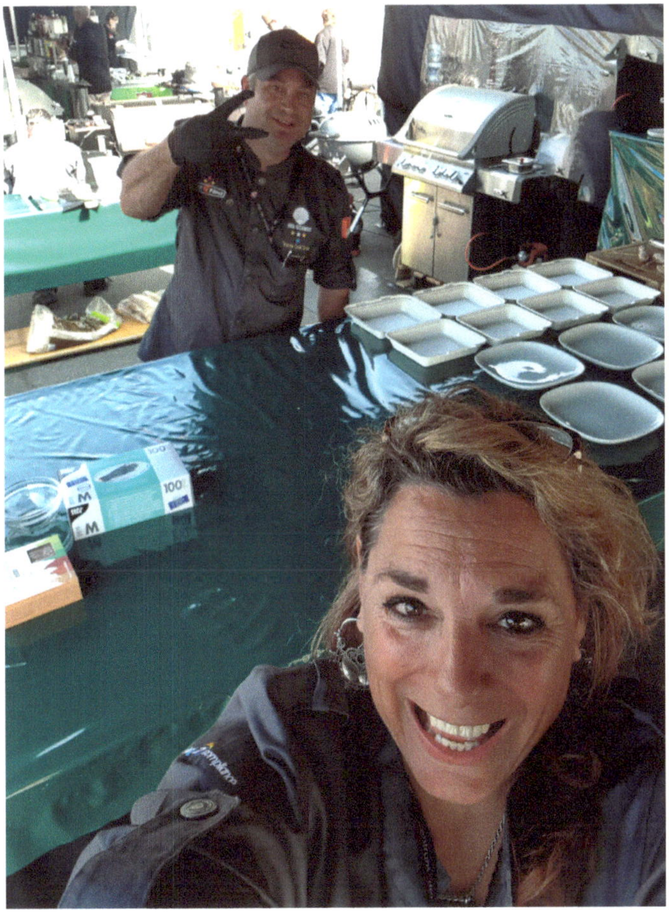

KARMA COOK

THE GOOD WILL OF GREAT FOOD

Follow us @ Facebook: Karma Cook

7

Spices, Rubs & Sauces

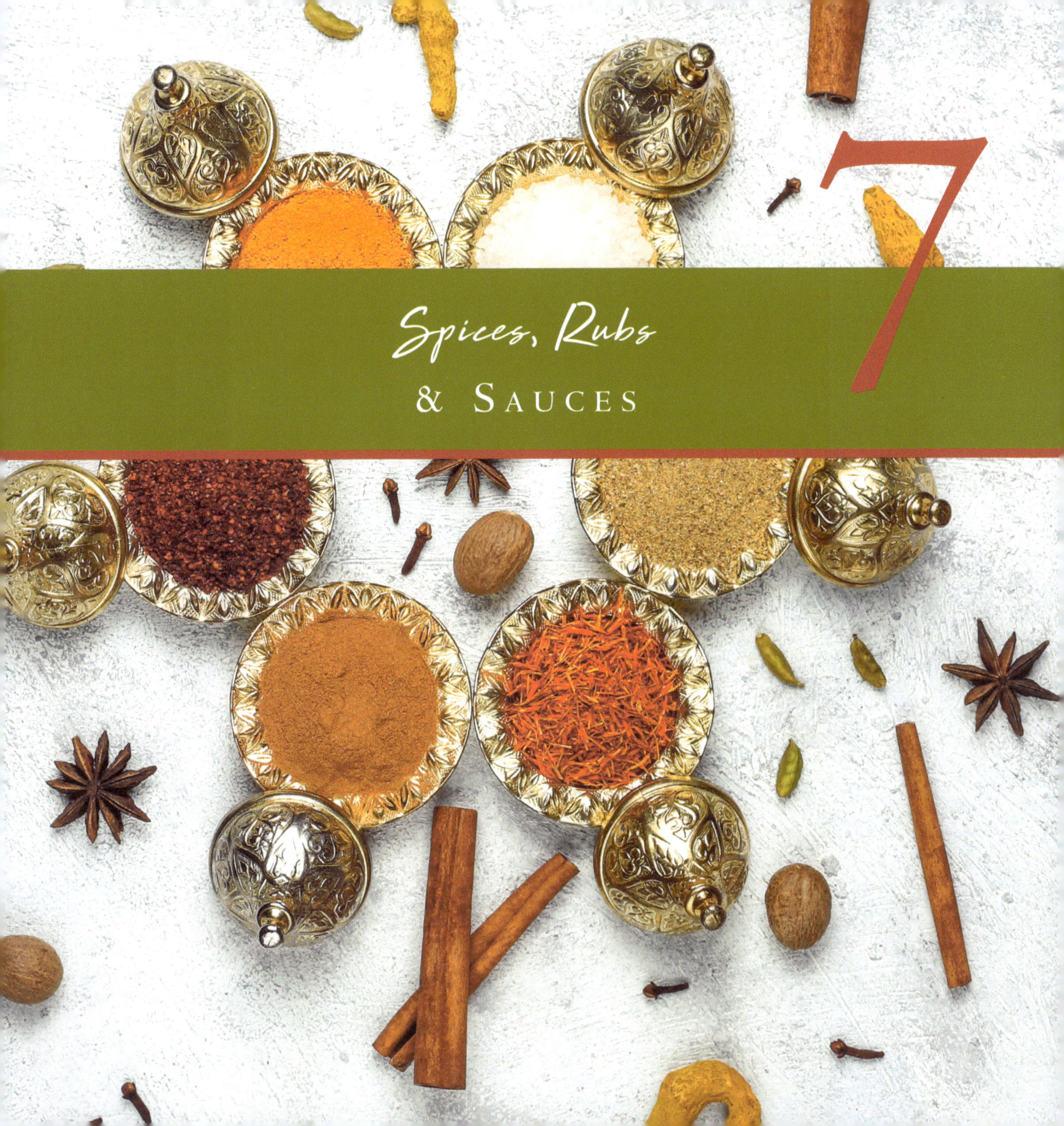

DF GF V

Blend of Herbs

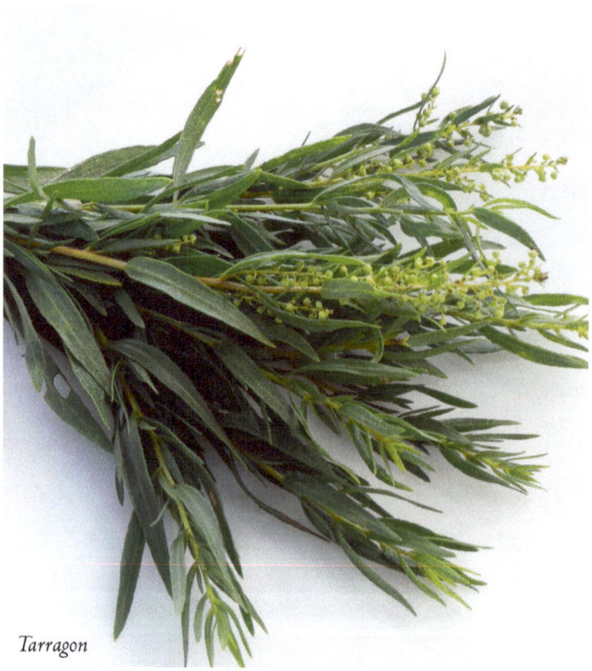

Tarragon

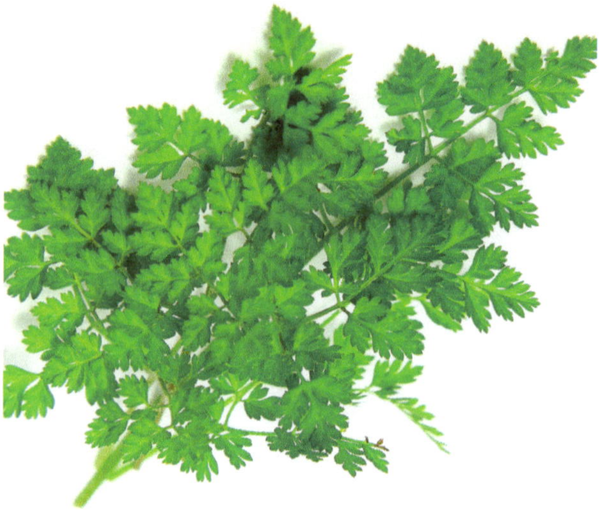

Chervil

Typically used in grilled meats, omelets and marinades, this blend of herbs is a French favorite. After spending much time in France, some of these tastes have stuck with me and bring back childhood memories and flavors.

You can also mix those in with butter, cream cheese, and mayonnaise to create a delightful spread for sandwiches and hors d'oeuvres.

1 sprig of fresh parsley	or	½ tsp. dried parsley flakes
1 sprig of fresh tarragon		¼ tsp. dried tarragon
1 sprig of fresh chervil		¼ tsp. dried chervil
1 fresh chive, chopped		

*Chervil is a French herb, related to parsley with a very delicate flavor.

Bouquet Garni – The Classic

Having spent part of my life with the French part of my family, many of the tastes and habits have carried over to my cooking. One of those is this French seasoning mix that gives a wonderful flavor to dishes. It is classically used for stews and other types of slow cooked meals. It also helps give depth to bean casseroles.

Typically, you would tie the sprigs of these fresh herbs together in a bouquet with cooking string or make a sachet with cheesecloth and then immerse them into your pot. Remove the herb bundle once the food is done cooking. Alternatively you can sprinkle the dried loose herbs in your pot while cooking.

3	sprigs of fresh parsley	or	1	tsp. dried parsley flakes
1	sprig of fresh thyme		¼	tsp. dried thyme
1	fresh bay leaf		1	dry bay leaf

Optional

1	sprig celery leaves	or	¼	tsp. celery seeds
1	sprig of fennel		⅛	tsp. dry fennel
1	sprig of marjoram		⅛	tsp. dry marjoram

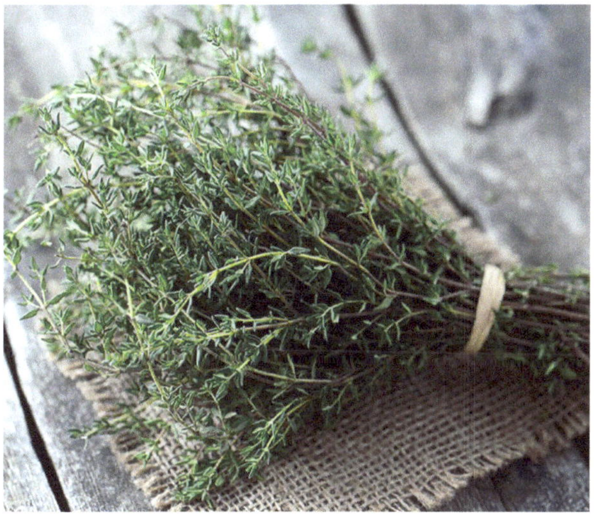

Thyme

Salt Mix For Grilled Veggies

Super easy and with so much flavor! When I am short on time, I will coarsely cut up some fresh veggies, like carrots, zucchini, and red onions and season them with this salt mix before roasting them in the oven.

- 2 tbsp. (Greek) sea salt
- 2 dry rosemary leaves
- ⅛ tsp. cracked pepper

Mix well and store in a small container for easy use when needed. When using to grill in the oven, first drizzle olive oil over veggies then sprinkle the salt mix.

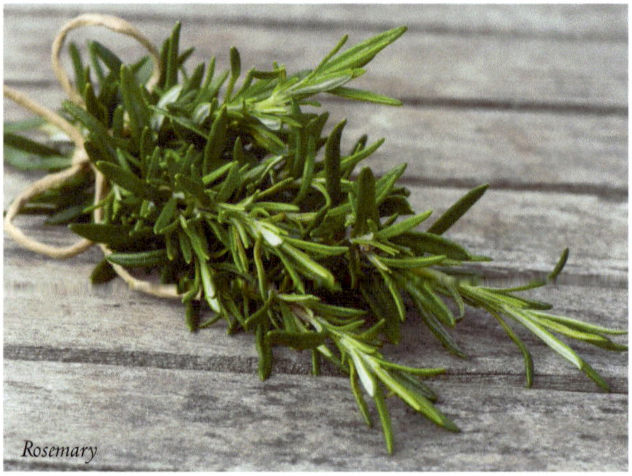

Rosemary

DF GF V

Season Salt - Homemade

Easy seasoning for burgers, skirt steak, chicken legs, kale chips and so much more.

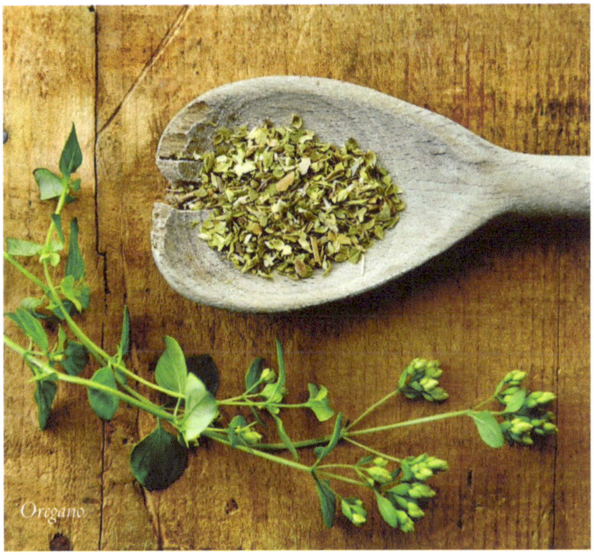

- 2 tbsp. (Greek) sea salt
- 1 tsp. paprika powder
- 1 tsp. raw sugar
- ½ tsp. celery powder
- ½ tsp. Greek oregano
- ⅛ tsp. cracked pepper
- ⅛ tsp. turmeric powder

Mix well and store in a sprinkling container for easy use when needed.

GF V

Spicy Chicken Rub

My husband makes the most amazing rubs and spices that result in scrumptious briskets, beef jerky and other delicious meats. I wanted to try my hand at a rub and came up with this mix for spicy chicken. You could either cook it on the grill on in the oven in a slow bake and then give it five minutes under broil to form a crust.

1	tbsp. sea salt
1	tbsp. ground black pepper
1	tbsp. ground cayenne pepper (adjust per your taste)
3	tbsp. paprika
2	tbsp. garlic powder
1 ½	tbsp. onion powder
1	tsp. Greek Oregano
⅛	tsp. Greek thyme

Place all ingredients in a wooden mortar and mix well with the pestle until all ingredients are powdered. You might get a bit more rub than you need depending on how heavy you like to sprinkle it on. If so, just save the rest for another time in a sealed glass container.

Take your chicken breasts and dry well with some paper towels. Take some coconut oil (warmed if in solid form) and baste all sides of the chicken breast. Then sprinkle on your rub generously using your fingers or a brush to make sure it is evenly spread. Place your chicken on a metal grill or a broiler and bake pan to catch the juices. Bake to perfection depending on the size of your chicken breasts and then remove in a serving plate to rest. If using a broiler pan sprinkle accumulated juice on top of chicken and serve.

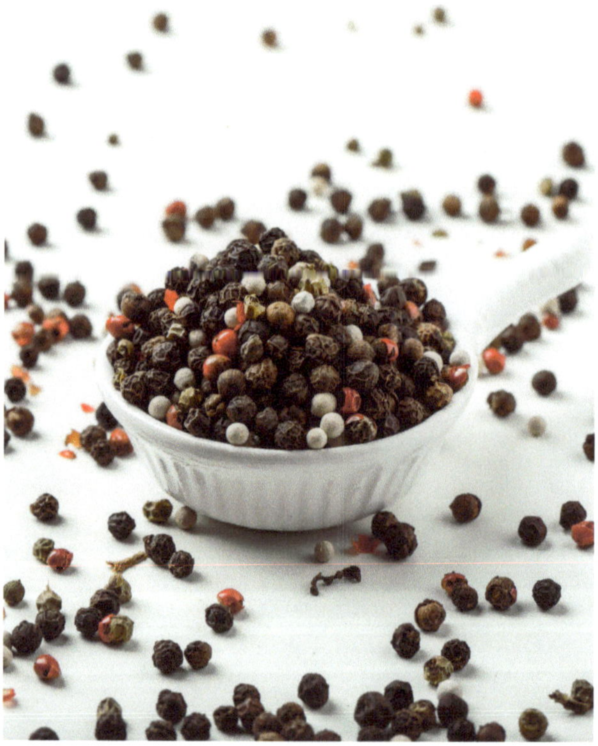

GF V

Sweet & Tangy

This blend is another quick and flavorful way to cook grilled veggies. Works as well in the oven as on the BBQ.

- 2 tbsps. (Greek) sea salt
- 1 tsp. cracked pepper
- 1 tsp. dried oregano
- ¼ cup olive oil drizzled over veggies
- 2 tbsps. balsamic vinegar

Drizzle olive oil and balsamic vinegar over cut up veggies and sprinkle with salt and pepper.

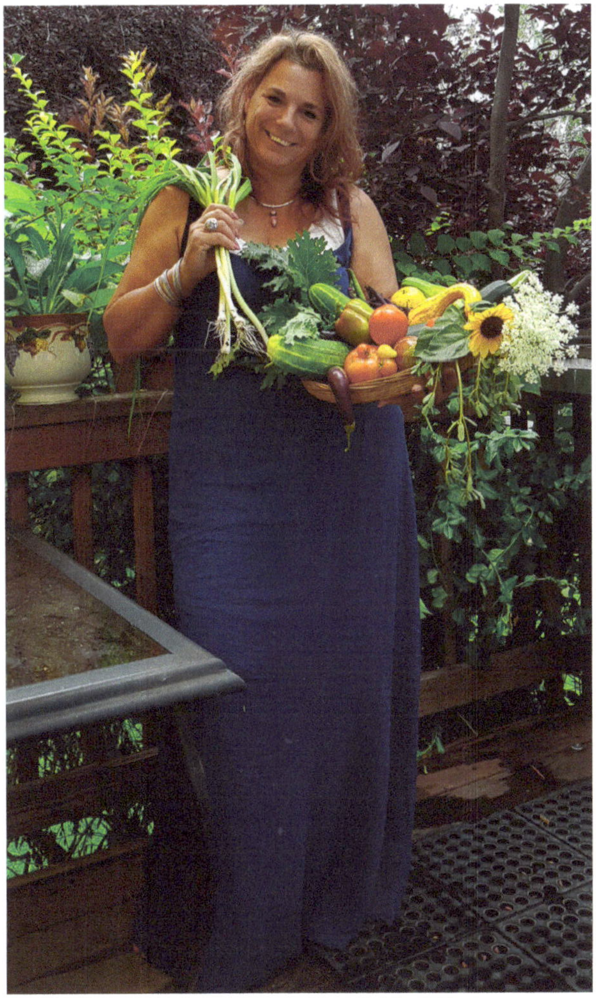

Za'atar Type Seasoning

This is one of my favorite mixes and I sprinkle it on so many dishes; from fish and chicken to lamb. It is also excellent as dipping oil when mixed with some olive oil. We often use it in the kitchen as it combines the basic Greek staple spices in one.

2	tbsp. Sumac
1 ½	tsp. toasted sesame seeds
1	tsp. sea salt
⅛	tsp. cumin
⅛	tsp. Greek Thyme
⅛	tsp. Greek Oregano
⅛	tsp. Greek marjoram

Mix well and store in a sprinkling container for easy use when needed. Sumac is a spice that originates from Turkey and in general the Middle East. It has a fruity, tart and lemony taste all at once and is a delicious addition to many Mediterranean dishes. The last three ingredients I generally bring back with me from Greece, but you can definitely find Greek herbs in most places that sell Mediterranean foods.

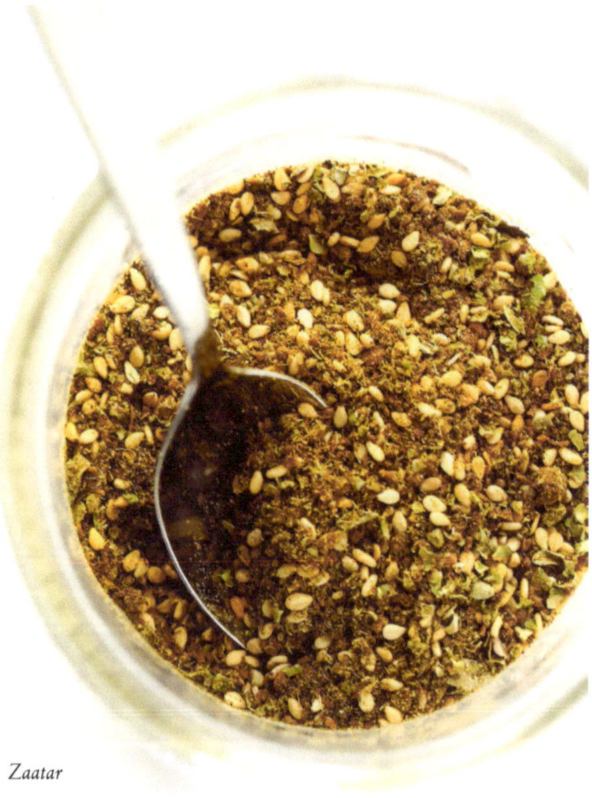

Zaatar

DF GF V

Avgolemono Sauce

Αυγολέμονο

This is a sauce found often in Greek dishes and made mostly from egg and lemons. The process is very sensitive and one needs to take care not to "cut" the eggs while mixing it with the hot broth. The lemony taste adds another level of depth into dishes such as chicken soup, stuffed cabbage leaves and stuffed grape leaves. You want to prepare this sauce right before your dish is ready and gently blend it into the food.

- 2-3 eggs at room temperature
- 2 large lemons, freshly juiced
- 2 cups of hot broth from meal

Take room temperature eggs and whisk until they become a pale yellow. While continuing to beat the eggs, drizzle in fresh lemon juice until it is well blended. Remove 2 cups of broth from the meal you are cooking, and gently drizzle it into the egg mixture, one ladle at a time while continuing to mix. You want to take care during this step to not go too fast or you risk cooking your eggs before they blend into the sauce.

When you have mixed in both cups of broth and sauce is now warm, slowly return Avgolemono sauce into the cooking pot and bring it to a very light boil.

Remove pot from fire and serve immediately

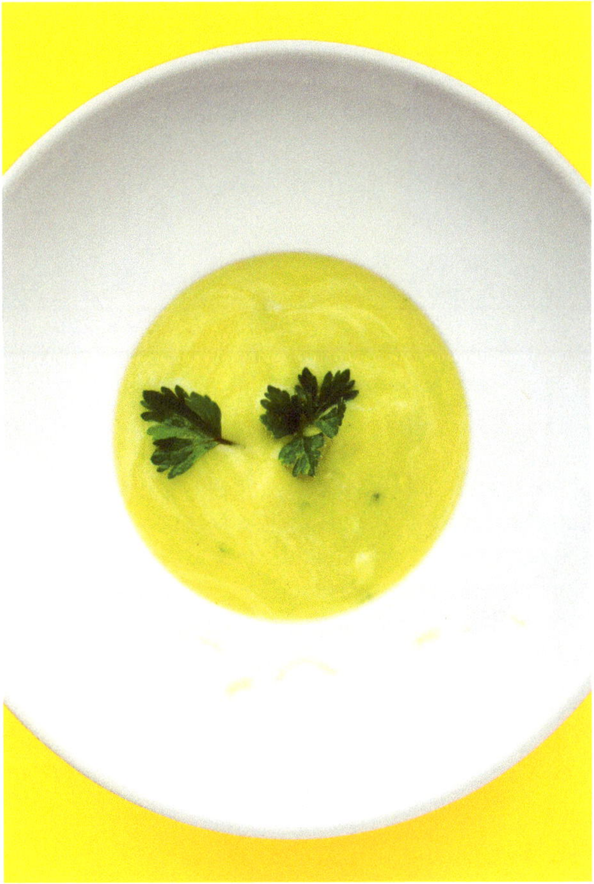

DF GF V

Balsamic Vinaigrette Dressing

Many people love this dressing, not only because of the tangy balsamic vinegar but because of its thick rewarding texture. It is so easy to make that it will quickly become one of your favorites.

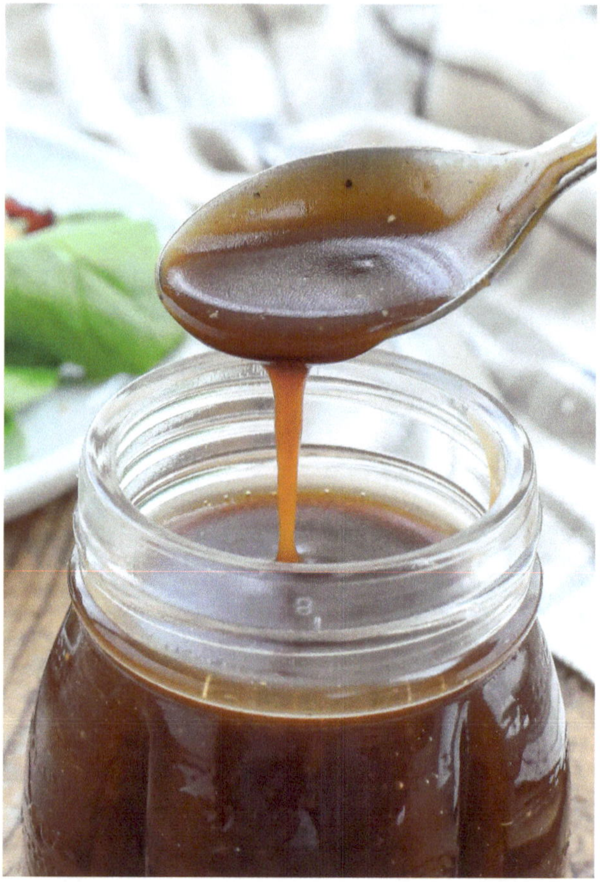

- ⅓ cup balsamic vinegar
- 1 tsp. honey
- 1 tsp. coconut aminos
- ⅛ tsp. Worcestershire sauce
- ½ cup Olive oil
- • Salt + Pepper to taste
- ½ tsp. xanthan gum powder

In this recipe the order of ingredients is essential in the preparation of the dressing. In a small container with a lid mix together vinegar and honey. Once dissolved, add aminos, Worcestershire sauce and drizzle in olive oil as you continue mixing and then add salt and pepper to taste.

Add the xantham gum a bit at a time and whisk with a fork or close container and shake vigorously untill dressing is emulsified and thickened. Serve over your favorite salad.

Serves 6 people *(All Seasons)*

DF GF V

Dijon Style Salad Dressing

One of my very favorite dressings and so easy to make. Sprinkle it over a green salad or a mix of cucumber and tomatoes. Also wonderful with raw cauliflower and green olive salad.

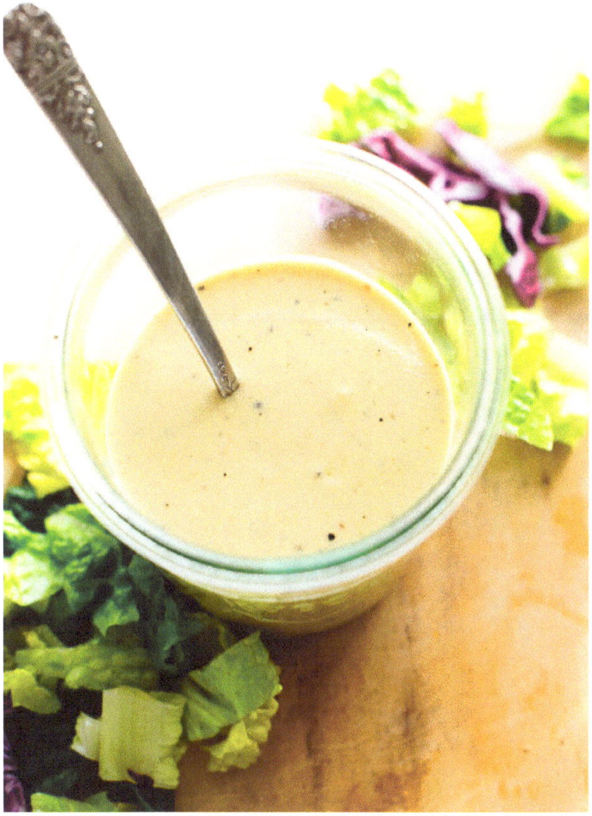

- ⅓ cup red wine vinegar
- ½ tsp. honey
- 1 tsp. Dijon mustard
- ½ cup Olive oil
- ½ tsp. salt
- • Pepper flakes (optional)

In this recipe the order of ingredients is essential in the preparation of the dressing. In a small container with a lid mix together vinegar and honey. Once dissolved, add mustard and mix well to dissolve. Slowly drizzle in olive oil, as you continue mixing, and then add salt and pepper to taste. Close container and shake vigorously untill dressing is emulsified. Serve over your favorite salad.

*You may adjust the quantity of the mustard according to your preference from stronger to milder tasting dressing.

Serves 4 people ***(All Seasons)***

Ladolemono Sauce

A very simple lemon and olive oil dressing, usually drizzled over freshly grilled fish.

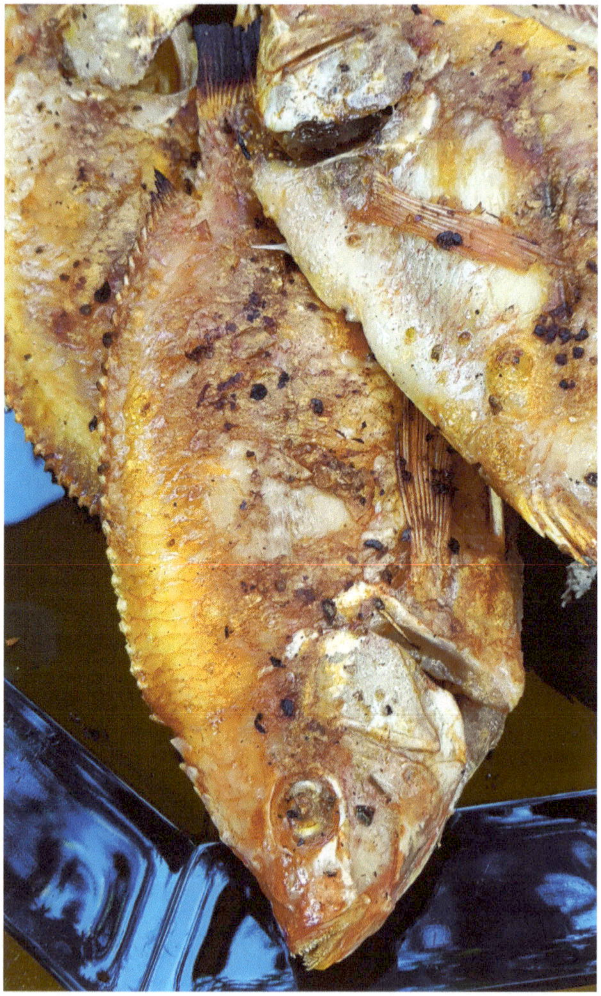

Ladolemono Sauce

- ¼ cup olive oil
- 1 lemon, juiced
- 1 tsp. dried oregano
- • Salt to taste

Drizzle lemon juice into olive oil, while continuously whisking and until well blended.

Add salt and serve over fish.

DF GF V

Light Salad Dressing

Any time you add apple cider vinegar to a dressing, it will be light and flavorful. In this recipe, the mustard adds a little tang and a bit more depth to the taste. Perfect for green salads and great with avocado as well.

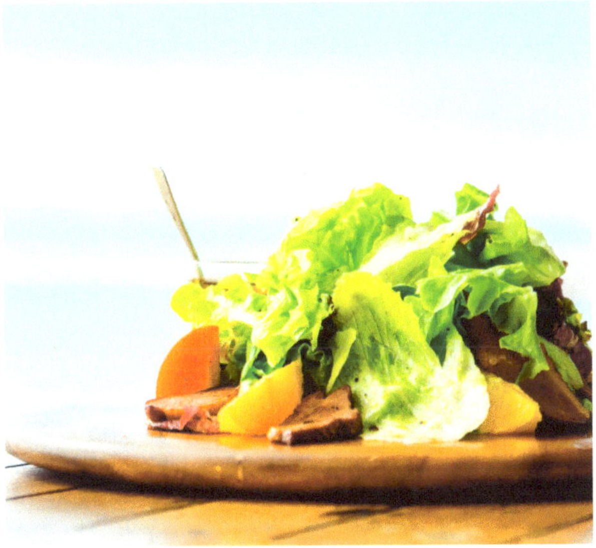

Dressing

- ⅓ cup apple cider vinegar
- 2 tbsps. seed mustard of your liking
- ½ cup olive oil
- • Salt + Pepper to taste

To blend this dressing, first pour vinegar in small container, then add seed mustard and mix until well dissolved. Add Olive oil, salt and pepper, mix well and drizzle over your favorite salad.

DF GF V

Taratur Sauce – Home Made

Simply Delicious and so easy to make. Use wonderful tahini sauce on meat dishes and light salads.

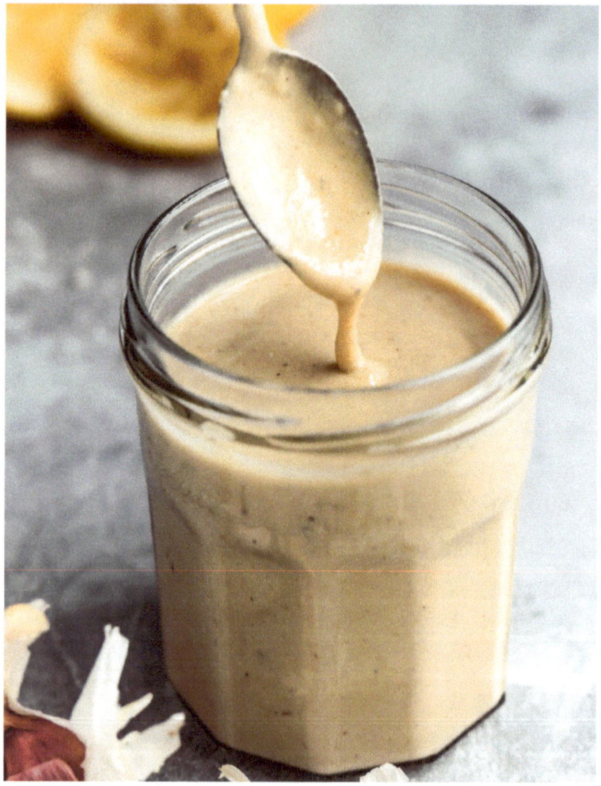

- 5 tbsps. Tahini (sesame seed paste)
- 5 tbsps. fresh squeezed lemon juice
- 3 tbsps. filtered water
- 1 garlic clove, minced (optional)
- ½ tsp salt or to taste

Tahini sauce is very thick and a bit difficul to break up in the beginnig. I like to slowly drizzle in the lemon juice while I mix it with a fork. Once that is well mixed you can slowly add the garlic and water, continue mixing untill it is well blended. Add the salt and it is ready to serve.

You can adjust the thickness of the sauce by how much water you add. If you like it more runny add a bit more water to your mix. But don't add too much or your sauce will loose its rich taste.

This sauce is wonderful with light salads and grilled meats, such as keftedes or kofta.

Serves 4 people *(All Seasons)*

DF GF V

Tartar Sauce – Home Made

Simply Delicious and so easy to make.

½	cup soy free Vegenaise
2	tbsp. olive oil
1	lemon, freshly squeezed
1	tbsp. relish
½	tsp salt
	• Pepper flakes (optional)

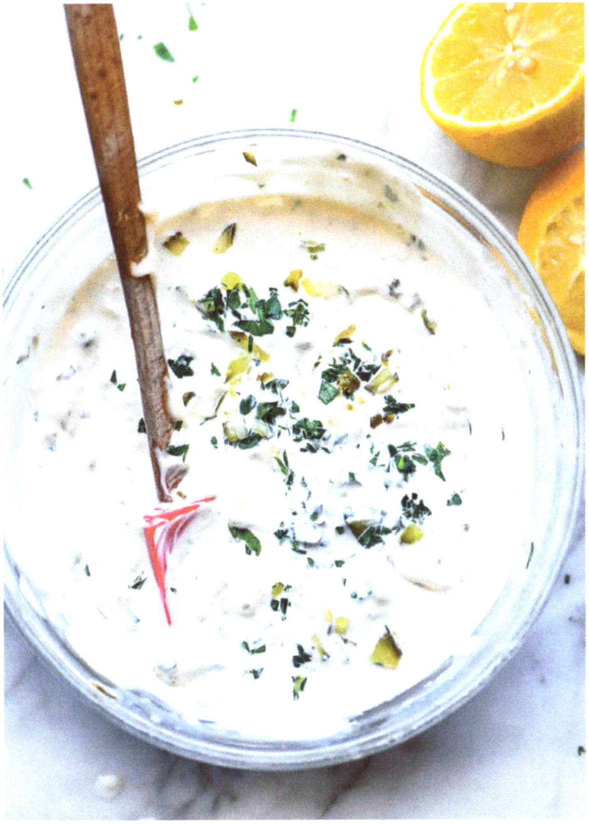

Vegenaise is a type of mayo sold in the stores, and in general, I prefer the one without soy in it. If you do not like the taste of mayonaise and its ingredients or it is too heavy for your tastebuds you might be pleasantly surprised by this product. Then again if you love mayo, feel free to substitute it in this sauce.

In a medium bowl mix vegenaise with olive oil until smooth. Add lemon juice and mix further. Add relish and salt and blend well.

This sauce is wonderful with fish sticks, schnitzel, and most breaded and fried recipes.

Serves 4 people *(All Seasons)*

GF V

TZATZIKI SAUCE

A sauce to dip just about everything in it if you are fond of yoghurt & garlic. There are many versions of tzatziki – this one being one of my favorites because I love the dill in it.

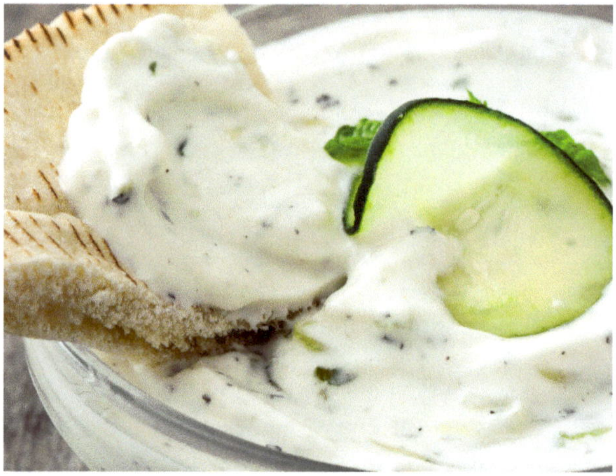

2	cups Greek strained yogurt
2	cloves of garlic, minced (per your preference)
½	cup grated, peeled cucumber (skin included)
1/12	tbsp. finely chopped dill or mint (your preference)
1 ½	tbsp. red wine vinegar or 1 teaspoon lemon juice
1	tbsp. Greek olive oil
	• Salt to taste

Tzatziki: Wash and grate cucumber whole and let sit in a colander for a while (at least two hours). Then squeeze excess moisture from the batch by either squeezing out small batches between your hands or pushing it through a sieve. In a small bowl, mix yogurt, minced garlic, herbs, cucumber and vinegar/lemon juice. Stir in olive oil. Add salt to taste and keep in fridge until ready to eat. It will generally keep about 2 weeks in the fridge but does become watery after a while.

Serves 8 people ***(Summer, Autumn)***

Pair with: Cut up crunchy veggies - carrots, celery, jicama root - or serve with pitta bread wedges. Also great with vegetable fritters, or served next to meat dishes.

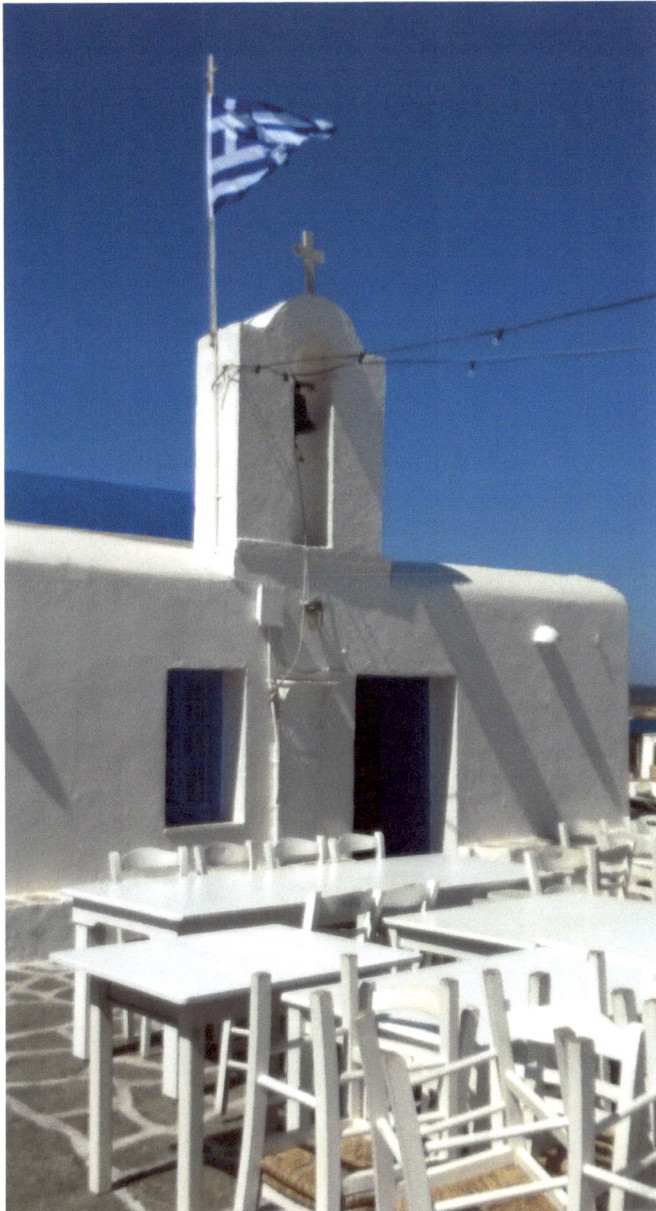

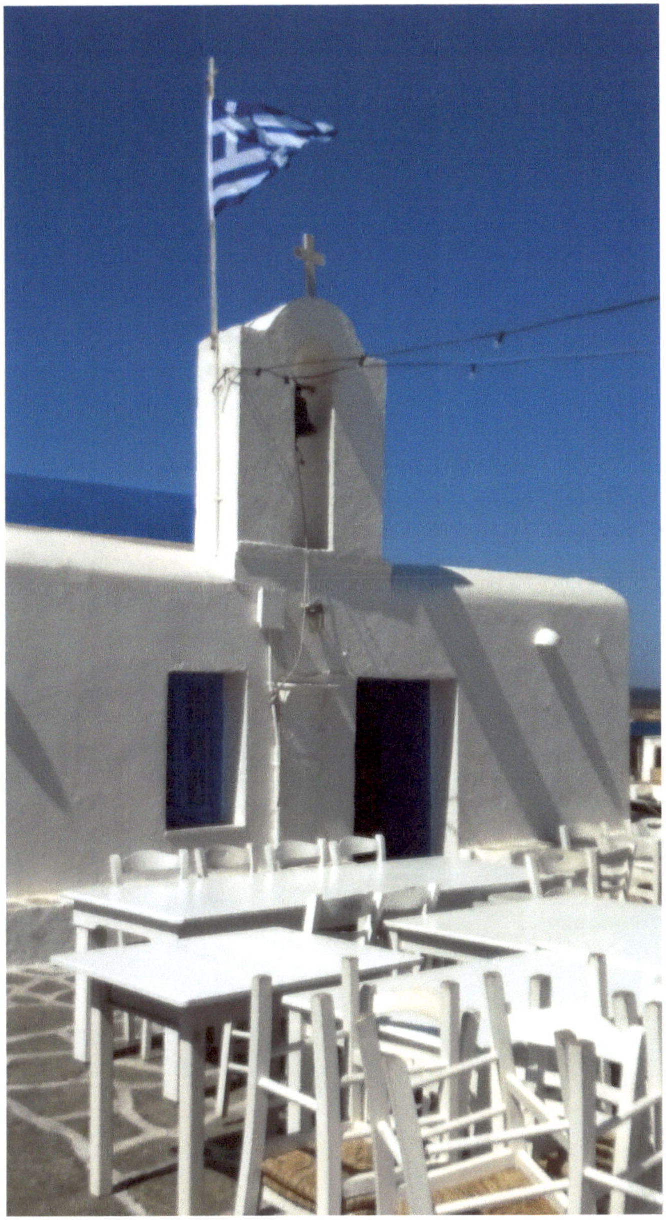

Rarely do I buy a salad dressing from the store as I can whip up my own creations that the whole family enjoys. Besides, most dressings on the market have fillers and toxic ingredients and way too much sugar for my palette.

If you make it a habit to read the labels of some dressings, you might decide that you can make a healthier version at home.

Most of these dressings above are easy to make and this way are fresh each time to enjoy on your favorite meal.

Each of the salad recipes in this book also comes with a description of its own dressing so you can choose your favorite.

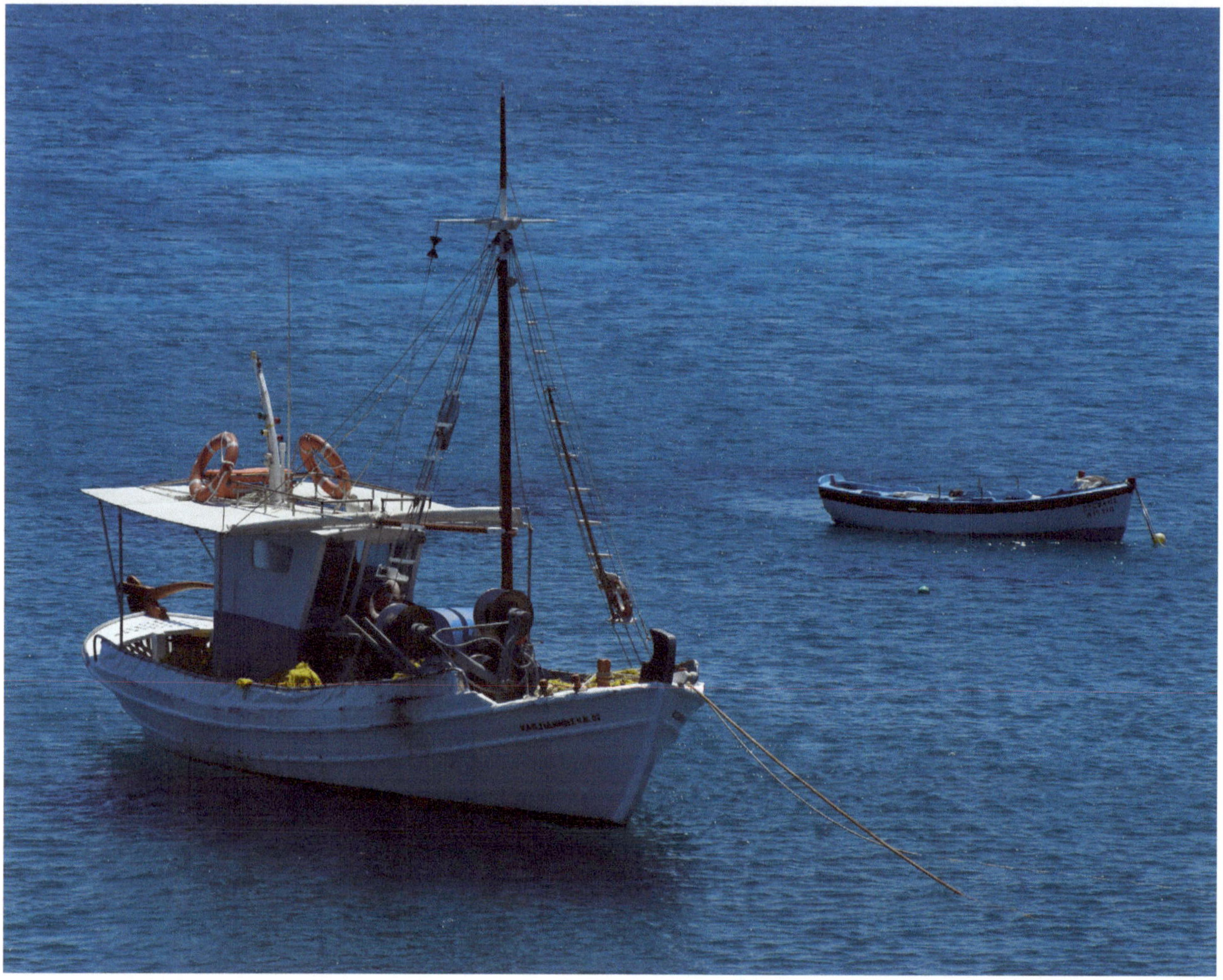

"Kaiki" - A typical Greek fishing boat

Acknowledgments

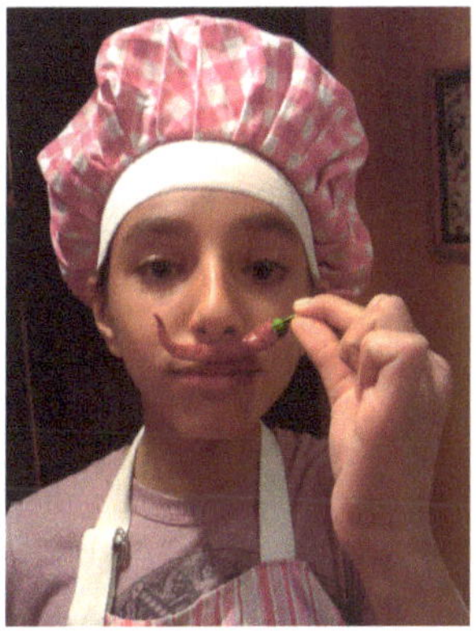

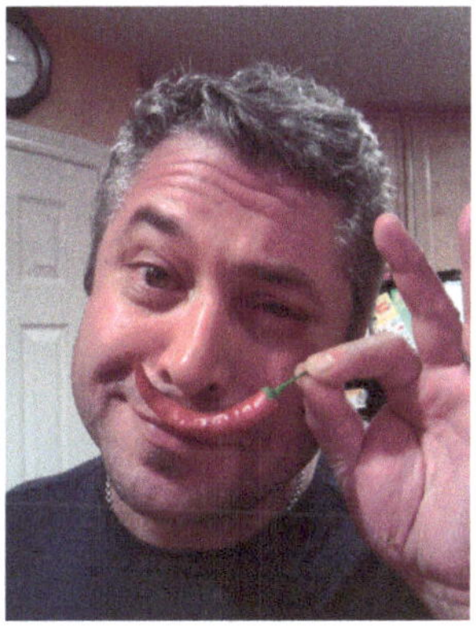

This compilation of information and recipes came from years spent in the kitchen next to my grandmothers, my mother, and my father, who lovingly prepared meals every day when I was growing up, and who tirelessly cooked up delicious creations that kept our tummies full and warmed our hearts. Even to this day, whenever I happen to visit home, I will be pleasantly surprised with my favorite dish upon my arrival!

I am grateful for the times spent together, for my loved ones always being there and especially for my mom who puts so much love into everything she does. To me this motherly nurturing, cooking delicious meals from scratch, picking vegetables from the garden and enjoying fresh picked seasonal fruit has been a way of life. Watching my mother tending to her organic farm, day in and day out, caring for her plants and animals, instilled in me a love for nature, that is with me to this day. I would like to express my gratitude to my family for those experiences and for everyone I grew up with and around. They were all an integral part of my growing up and the reason why I love to cook, grow a garden and share my knowledge with the world today.

Much of my gratitude goes to my immediate family and especially my husband, who shares the passion for cooking and who has spent many hours alongside me, prepping, and creating, teaching and catering events. His creativity and input have been an essential part of my evolving culinary world. Sharing his nurturing and caring ways has been essential in the preparation and creation of the meals we serve on our family table. And to our beautiful kids who never cease to amaze me with their braveness in the kitchen, trying new recipes and ideas that they are inspired with. They sometimes surprise us with a delicious home cooked meal or a sweet treat, beautiful raw vegetable creations and smoothies.

A big thank you also goes out to many friends that were willing to put some of these recipes to the test for themselves and provide valuable feedback. Also, to those who helped with proofreading, editing, designing and tirelessly going over this book again and again.

This creation has been a group effort. As they say, *it takes a village to raise a child* – and a community to bring a cookbook to completion. Thank you to all for being part of our extended Mediterranean Family!

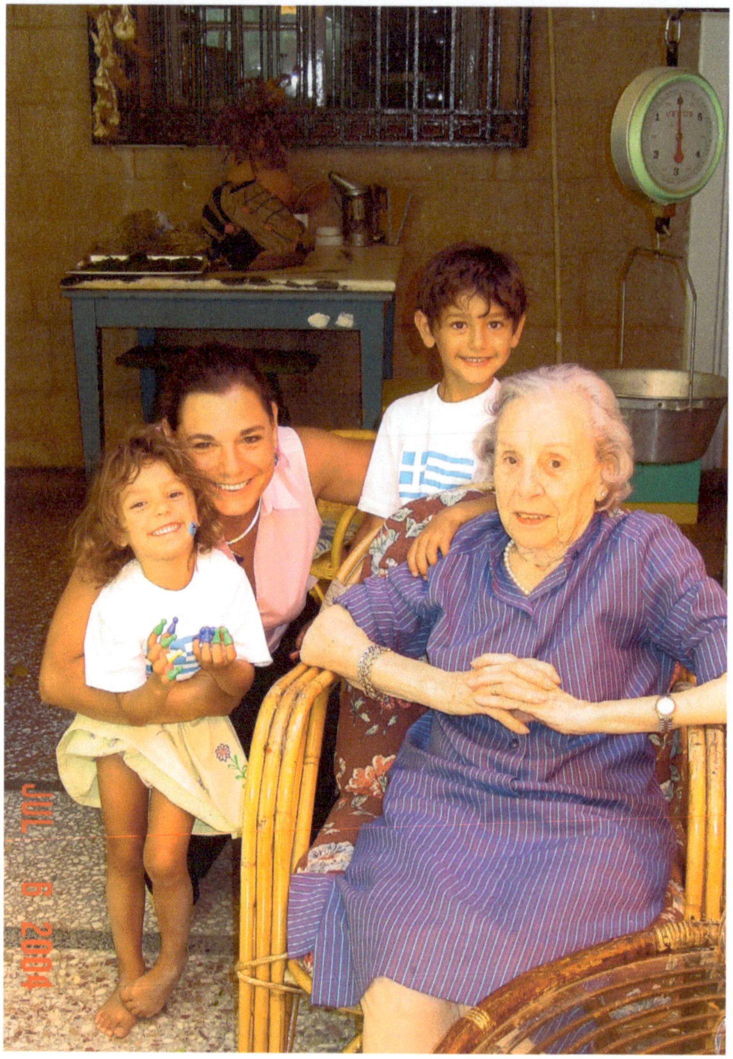

With great Grandma

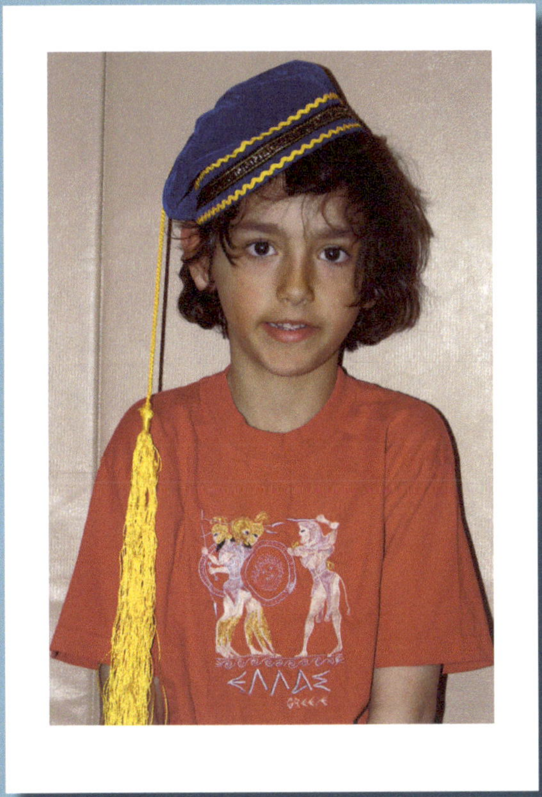

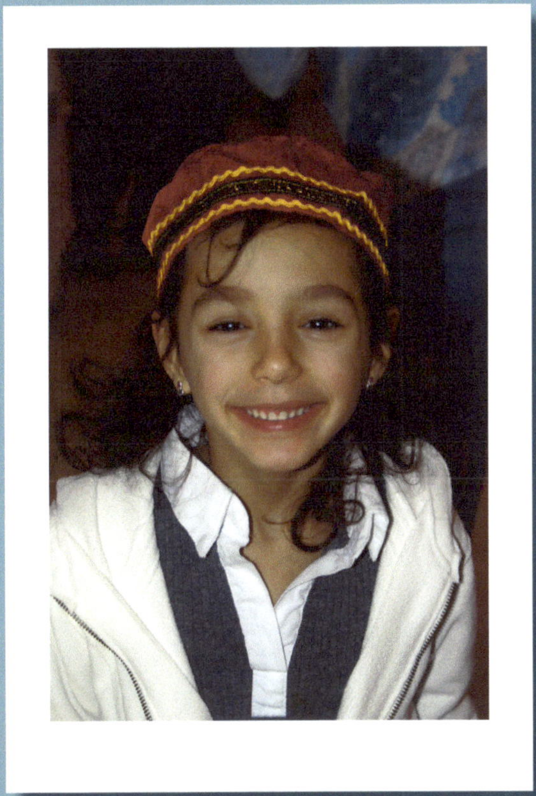

My kiddos

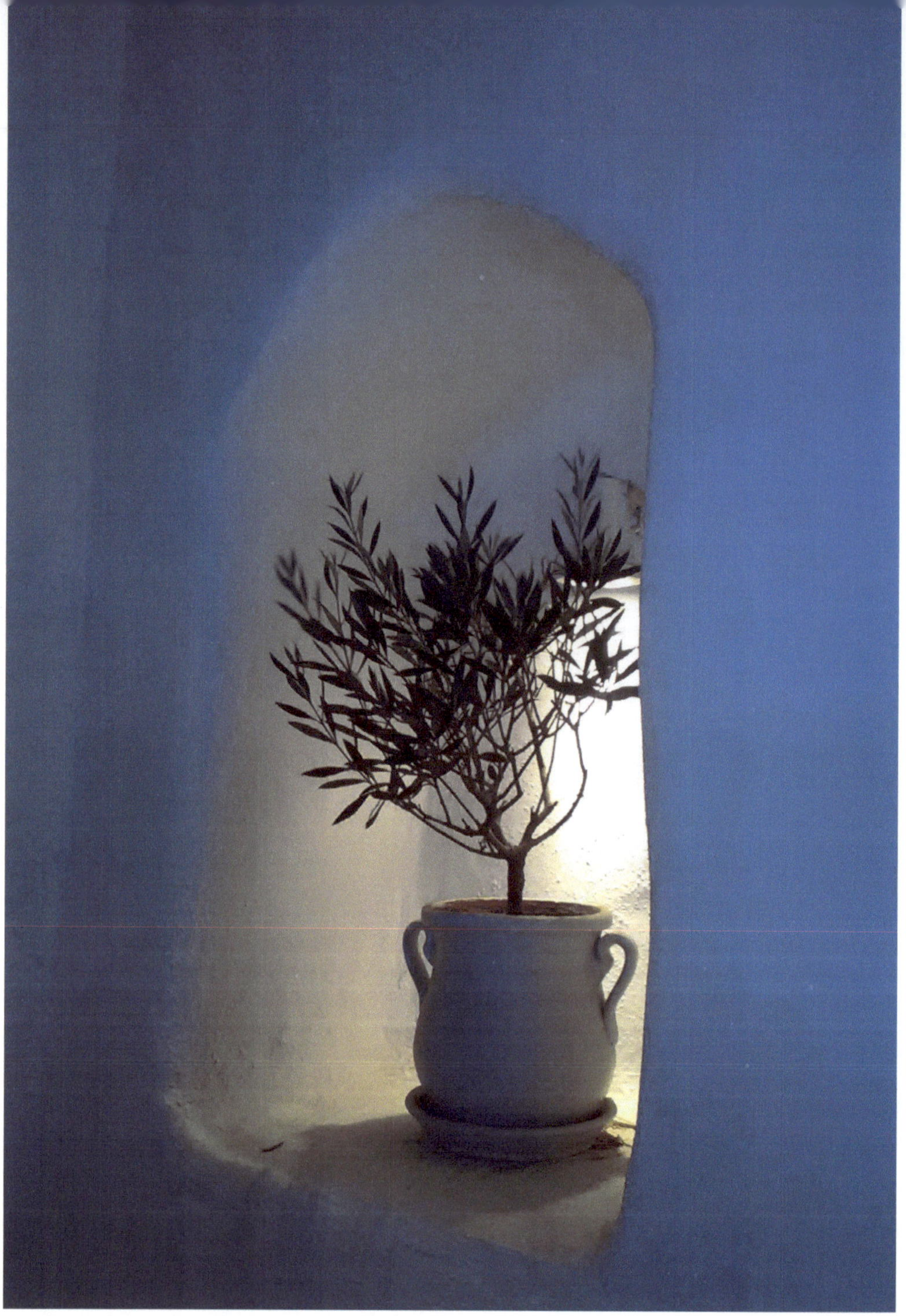

Recipe Index

Recipe Index

Recipe Index

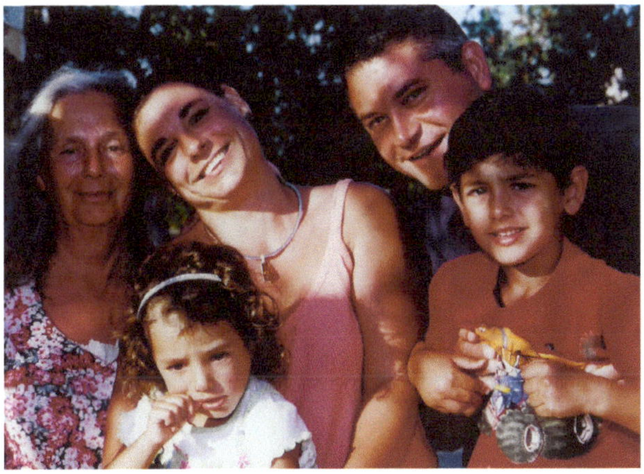

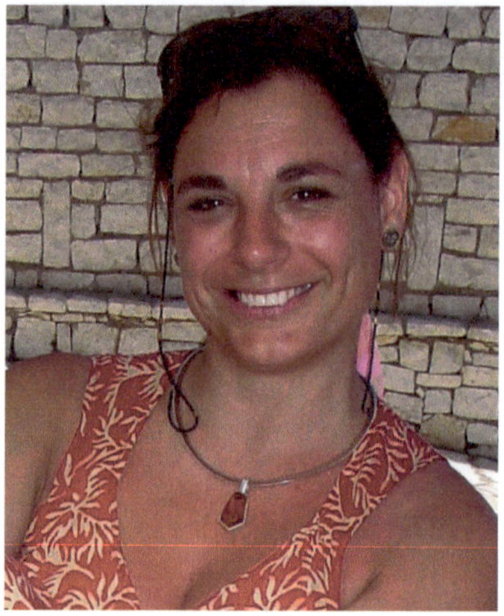

Corinna P. Kromer

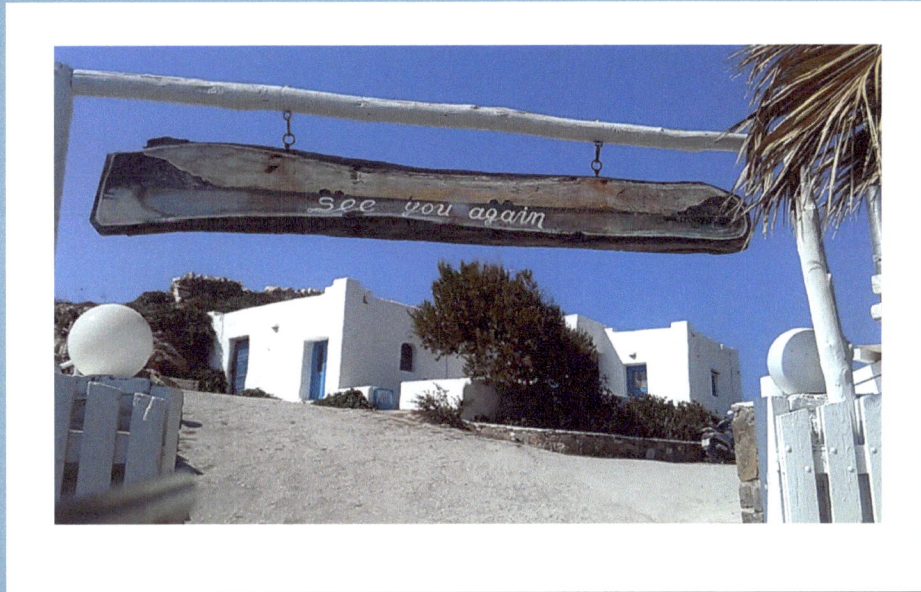

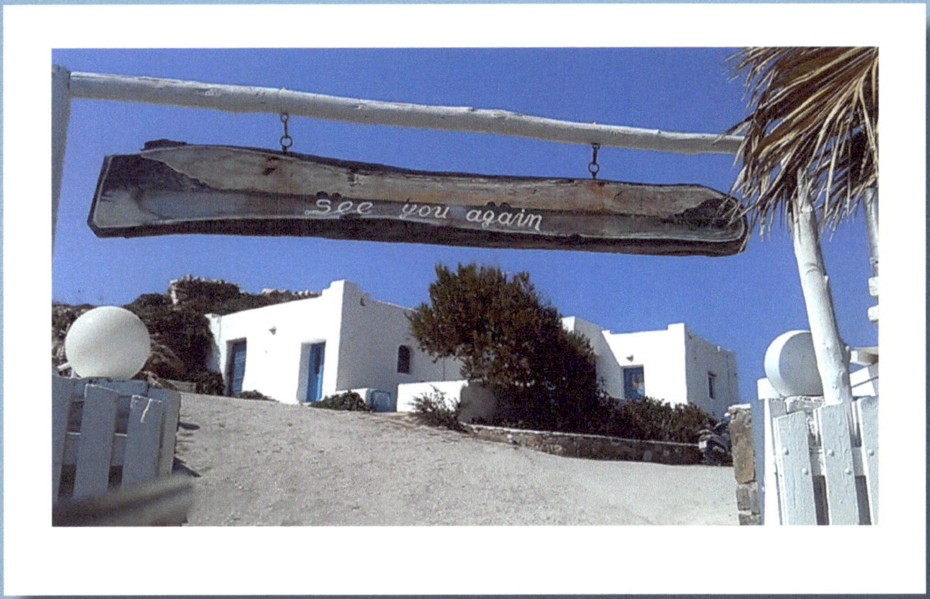

BON APPETIT!

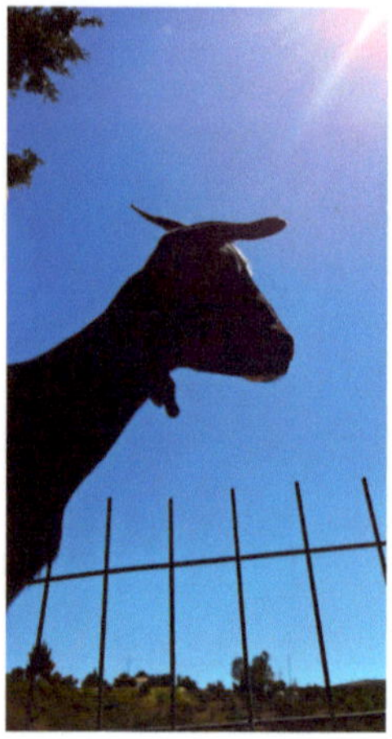

Colorado, 2021

www.ingramcontent.com/pod-product-compliance
Lightning Source LLC
Chambersburg PA
CBHW042022090426
42811CB00016B/1710
* 9 7 8 0 9 8 5 7 0 5 7 7 0 *